Medical Discourse
and
Systemic Frames of Comprehension

Ronald J. Chenail

Institute for Systemic Therapy
Nova University

Volume XLII in the Series
ADVANCES IN DISCOURSE PROCESSES
Roy O. Freedle, Editor

ABLEX PUBLISHING CORPORATION
NORWOOD, NEW JERSEY

Library of Congress Cataloging-in-Publication Data

Chenail, Ronald J.
Medical discourse and systematic frames of comprehension / by Ronald J. Chenail.
p. cm. -- (Advances in discourse processes ; v. 42)
Includes bibliographical references and index.
ISBN (invalid) 0-89391-709-9 (cl)
1. Discourse analysis. 2. Communication in medicine. I. Title. II. Series.
[DNLM: 1. Communication. 2. Cognition. 3. Physician-Patient Relations. W 62 C518m]
P302.C44 1990
610'.14--dc20
DNLM/DLC 90-14418
for Library of Congress CIP

Printed in the United States of America.

Ablex Publishing Corporation
355 Chestnut Street
Norwood, New Jersey 07648

With Jan

Table of Contents

Preface to the Series

Roy O. Freedle

Series Editor

This series of volumes provides a forum for the cross-fertilization of ideas from a diverse number of disciplines, all of which share a common interest in discourse—be it prose comprehension and recall, dialogue analysis, text grammar construction, computer simulation of natural language, cross-cultural comparisons of communicative competence or other related topics. The problems posed by multisentence contexts and the methods required to investigate them, while not always unique to discourse, are still sufficiently distinct as to benefit from the organized model of scientific interaction made possible by this series.

Scholars working in the discourse area from the perspective of sociolinguistics, psycholinguistics, ethnomethodology and the sociology of language, educational psychology (e.g., teacher-student interaction), the philosophy of language, computational linguistics, and related subareas are invited to submit manuscripts of monograph or book length to the series editor. Edited collections of original papers resulting from conferences will also be considered.

Volumes in the Series

Vol. I.	Discourse Production and Comprehension. Roy O. Freedle (Ed.), 1977.
Vol. II.	New Directions in Discourse Processing. Roy O Freedle (Ed.), 1979.
Vol. III.	The Pear Stories: Cognitive, Cultural, and Linguistic Aspects of Narrative Production. Wallace L. Chafe (Ed.), 1980.
Vol. IV.	Text, Discourse, and Process: Toward a Multidisciplinary Science of Texts. Robert de Beaugrande, 1980.

Vol. V. Ethonography and Language in Educational Settings. Judith Green & Cynthia Wallat (Eds.), 1981.
Vol. VI. Latino Language and Communicative Behavior. Richard P. Duran (Ed.), 1981.
Vol. VII. Narrative, Literacy and Face in Interethnic Communication. Ron Scollon & Suzanne Scollon, 1981.
Vol. VIII. Linguistics and the Professions. Robert J. DiPietro (Ed.), 1982.
Vol. IX. Spoken and Written Language: Exploring Orality and Literacy. Deborah Tannen (Ed.), 1982.
Vol. X. Developmental Issues in Discourse. Jonathan Fine & Roy O. Freedle (Eds.), 1983.
Vol. XI. Text Production: Toward a Science of Composition. Robert de Beaugrande, 1984.
Vol. XII. Coherence in Spoken and Written Discourse. Deborah Tannen (Ed.), 1984.
Vol. XIII. The Development of Oral and Written Language in Social Contexts. Anthony D. Pellegrini & Thomas D. Yawkey (Eds.), 1984.
Vol. XIV. What People Say They Do With Words. Jef Verschueren, 1985.
Vol. XV. Systemic Perspectives on Discourse, Volume 1: Selected Theoretical Papers from the 9th International Systemic Workshop. James D. Benson & William S. Greaves (Eds.), 1985.
Vol. XVI. Systemic Perspectives on Discourse, Volume 2: Selected Applied Papers from the 9th International Systemic Workshop. James D. Benson & William S. Greaves (Eds.), 1985.
Vol. XVII. Structures and Procedures of Implicit Knowledge. Arthur C. Graesser & Leslie F. Clark, 1985.
Vol. XVIII. Contexts of Reading. Carolyn N. Hedley & Anthony N. Baratta (Eds.), 1985.
Vol. XIX. Discourse and Institutional Authority: Medicine, Education, and Law. Sue Fisher & Alexandra Dundas Todd (Eds.), 1986.
Vol. XX. Evidentiality: The Linguistic Coding of Epistemology. Wallace Chafe & Johanna Nichols (Eds.), 1986.
Vol. XXI. The Acquisition of Literacy: Ethnographic Perspectives. Bambi B. Schieffelin & Perry Gilmore (Eds.), 1986.
Vol. XXII. Cognitive and Linguistic Analyses of Test Performance. Roy O. Freedle & Richard P. Duran (Eds.), 1987.
Vol. XXIII. Linguistic Action: Some Empirical-Conceptual Studies. Jef Verschueren (Ed.), 1987.
Vol. XXIV. Text and Epistemology. William Frawley, 1987.
Vol. XXV. Second Language Discourse: A Textbook of Current Research. Jonathan Fine (Ed.), 1988.
Vol. XXVI. Systemic Functional Approaches to Discourse. James D. Benson & William S. Greaves (Eds.), 1988.
Vol. XXVII. Language Development: Learning Language, Learning Culture. Ruqaiya Hasan & James Martin (Eds.), 1989.
Vol. XXVIII. Multiple Perspective Analyses of Classroom Discourse. Judith L. Green & Judith O. Harker (Eds.), 1988.
Vol. XXIX. Linguistics in Context: Connecting Observation and Understanding. Deborah Tannen (Ed.), 1988.
Vol. XXX. Gender and Discourse: The Power of Talk. Alexandra D. Todd & Sue Fisher (Eds.), 1988.

Acknowledgments

My gratitude goes to the families who volunteered a little bit of their life for this project. I know it was difficult for parents to talk about their child's heart and I hope that their stories will be helpful to other families who will have to deal with a child who has been diagnosed as having a heart murmur.

I would like to thank the doctors, staff, and administration of Department of Pediatrics at the Texas Tech University Health Sciences Center (TTUHSC) for their encouragement and financial support for this project. I would especially like to give credit to Dr. Joon M. Park for his guidance in this research.

Also, I would like to recognize the contributions made to this project by my colleagues: Paul Douthit, Jerry Gale, and Jeff Stormberg. From the initial planning sessions of the project at TTUHSC, to the final drafts of this document, their contributions have been immense, and greatly appreciated. I would also like to acknowledge Douglas Flemons for his assistance and friendship, Dr. Monte Bobele for his initiative in paving the way for this research, Dr. Roy O. Freedle for his support and helpful criticism of this book, and the fine people at Ablex Publishing Corporation, including Barbara Bernstein and Carol Davidson, who helped with the final preparations of this work.

I would like to thank Dr. John M. Flynn for his support and guidance, not only for his help with this research, but also for his leadership as Dean of the School of Social Sciences at Nova University.

I would also like to acknowledge Dr. Bud Morris' contributions to this project. I greatly respect his work, his ideas, and his integrity. In his own quiet way, Bud has had a tremendous influence on my development as a researcher and as a person.

I owe Dr. Brad Keeney more than words could ever express. He has always been an inspiration to me with his words, ideas, and friendship. I know that my work and my life have benefited from having had the opportunity to be with Brad, and for that I am thankful.

I would like to thank my family for their support and love. My mother has always been there for me, and her belief in me has never wavered. George and Michelle are the two finest children a father could ever want. And finally, I would like to share this moment with my wife, Jan. Our relationship is what I prize most in life and I am forever grateful for all that she is.

SOURCES

Sections of Chapters 1, 3, and 4 in this book were previously published by Lawrence Erlbaum Associates, Inc., in their journal *Health Communication*, and the sections are reprinted here by the permission of the publishers.

Chenail, R. J., Douthit, P. E., Gale, J. E., Stormberg, J. L., Morris, G. H., Park, J. M., Sridaromont, S., & Schmer, V. (1990). "It's probably nothing serious, but. . .": Parents' interpretation of referral to pediatric cardiologists. *Health Communication, 2 (3), 165-187.*

Chapter 1
Heartfelt Stories

INTRODUCTION

A promising development in the nature of inquiry has been the adoption of a stance or posture (Schumacher, 1989) known as the narrative paradigm (see Fisher, 1987, 1989; Ricoeur, 1981; Spence, 1982, 1987): "a conceptual framework, like dramatism, for understanding human decision, discourse, and action" (Fisher, 1989, p. 55). Human communication, from this perspective, is understood as story telling, wherein people narrate their experiences of past and current events.

> If the narrative paradigm celebrates anything, it celebrates human beings, and it does this by reaffirming their nature as storytellers. It affirms that narration as individuated form and as genre—like other individuated forms (such as argument) and genre (such as argumentation)—are expressive of good reasons, if viewed rhetorically. And when they are so experienced, they are constitutive of people, community, and the world. (Fisher, 1989, p. 56)

Central to this world view is the relationship between narrativity and historicity or in other words, the unfolding of "the description and redescription of our historical condition" (Ricoeur, 1981, p. 274). The narrative paradigm focuses on both the historical event and the retelling of said event. Such a perspective makes possible both a fictional history and a historical fiction. Ricoeur (1981, p. 274) reminds us of "the fundamental and radical fact that we make history, that we are immersed in history, that we are historical beings." As careful observers and storytellers, we dutifully acknowledge and record our experiences, and communicate these personal histories in our written and spoken discourse.

These stories have both a chronological and a nonchronological dimension (Ricoeur, 1981, p. 278). The chronological speaks to the episodic nature of narrative: stories and lives consist of temporal events. The nonchronological addresses the semantic nature of narratives: People as story tellers "also construct meaningful totalities out of scattered events" or "attempt to 'grasp together' successive events" in order "to exact a configuration from a succession" (Ricoeur, 1981, p. 278).

Implicit in the multidimensional quality of the narrative paradigm is the avoidance of embracing either a discovery of facts orientation (an accent on historicity) or a construction of fiction stance (an emphasis on narrativity); the predominance of one might lead to the preclusion of the other. By concentrating on the relationship between history and fiction, the narrative paradigm proposes an inquiry which is interpretive in nature and practice. Research from this perspective involves the telling and retelling of stories, or the interpretations of interpretations. The investigator interprets the oral or written stories of the storytellers in order to represent the stories in written or oral form. The represented stories, in turn, are reinterpreted by a reader to form new and different stories. In its most simplest form, a narrative-informed researcher is interested in studying and retelling other people's storytelling.

This text represents an attempt to conduct inquiry from a narrative perspective. It is the retelling of families' stories focusing on one of the most important subjects to us as human beings—the heart. " 'Heart,' after 'man,' 'god,' 'world,' 'life,' and the heart's corollary, 'love,' is the subject of more quotes in Bartlett's *Familiar Quotations* than any other reference. No part of us has been more problematic, more pondered, or poeticized" (Siebert, 1990, p. 56). The plot of each families' tale involves a child being referred to a pediatric cardiologist for the purpose of having a suspected innocent heart murmur examined. Discourse is collected, texts are constructed, and the task of the researcher is to interpret these stories of particularity and to re-present the participants' talk as they partake in the referral process and attempt to derive meaning from their heartfelt experiences. The next step in the inquiry process involves the reader, who now has the fourfold task of (a) interpreting the interpretations, (b) judging the acceptability of the conclusions drawn in this text (Ricoeur, 1981, p. 277), (c) critically considering this mode of inquiry (see Nelson, Megill, & McCloskey, 1988), one based upon a "literary approach to rhetoric [that] has begun to re-emerge with the communication field's approach, on the common ground of narrativity, metaphor, and figuration" (Lyne, 1985, p. 65), and (d) reading on.

MATTERS OF THE HEART

Professionals sometimes encounter situations in which they do not consider their expertise sufficient to handle and complete the matters at hand. When this happens, they refer clients to others who are better equipped, by virtue of specialized education and experience, to continue treatment or service. Many of these referrals may be both routine and unproblematic, but that is not necessarily the case. Not infrequently, the speech act of referral is interpreted to mean that something severe may be wrong. For instance, parents told that their child needs to see a specialist in learning disorders would have justifiable grounds in being concerned. The same goes for people referred to tax accountants, marriage counselors, or criminal attorneys.

When professionals reflect upon the process of referral, their attention is focused on such matters as the reasons the client or patient should see another professional, who should that other helper be, when shall the appointment be made, and so on. What seems to be ignored in this self-study is the essence of the referral itself: the talk. What transpires during the face-to-face interaction? Who says what to whom when and so forth.

Equally important, and also overlooked in the phenomenology of the referral, is the time after the referral, when the client or patient begins to create his or her understanding of the professional's words. Through conversations with family members, friends, other professional helpers, and themselves, people construct meaning for their experiences. Thus, one's perception of the referral consists of the act itself (the talk) and the subsequent considerations and reconsiderations of the initial act (the talk about the talk).

As in other professional arenas, medical specialization has advanced to the point in the United States that one doctor making a referral to another is a very common occurrence (e.g., Hansen, Bobula, Meyer, Kusher, & Pridham, 1987; Hansen, Brown, Sullivan, & Muhlbaier, 1982). "Referral of patients from one physician to another is essential to providing quality medical care" (Glenn, Lawler, & Hoerl, 1987, p. 1929), but there may be some drawbacks with the process. The interpretation of referral as portending something grave in the offing is unmistakably present and consequential in the case of referrals in the field of medicine. Of course, not just any referral may promote alarm. Alarm-generating cases seem to take place between a generalist (e.g., family or general practitioner) and a specialist, such as the pediatric cardiologist (Hersher, 1988; McNamara, 1987a, 1987b, 1988). Seemingly, alarm is provoked when referral is made to one whose specialty is a vital organ. As Hersher (1988) contends, the act of referral to a heart specialist "suggests that something is amiss with that most vital of body organs" (p. 587). As with referral by other professionals, the mere fact of referral for a potentially serious ailment may evoke the worry that the referral is not routine, not just a precaution, but rather that it is something about which to be seriously worried (McNamara, 1987a,

1987b, 1988). Indeed, ample medically-oriented literature has apprised physicians of the association of referral with worry on the part of the patients (e.g., Bergman & Stamm, 1967). Much of this literature concentrates on proper diagnosis and/or referral of heart murmurs (Gidding & Rosenthal, 1984; Goldfield, Neinstein, & Wohlgelernter, 1986).

One of the most important and also most common procedures asked of the primary care physician (e.g., pediatrician or family practitioner) is to correctly diagnose the innocent heart murmur (Paraskos, 1988). It is estimated that between 40 to 50 percent of the childhood population may have innocent heart murmurs (Bergman & Stamm, 1967; McNamara, 1987b). Murmur refers to that sound produced in the heart by normal, but high flow, velocity through the various valves in the heart (Paraskos, 1988). The murmur is described as being innocent if there is "no abnormal cardiovascular physiology and no structural defects in the heart and great vessels" (Paraskos, 1988, pp. 20–21); in simpler terms, if the murmur or sound heard by the physician "is not associated with any disease or abnormality of the heart" (McNamara, 1987a, p. 1), then the heart murmur is innocent or insignificant and should not cause any physical or developmental problems for the patient.

Besides the consideration of structural defects, there are additional factors involved which can make the diagnosis of innocent murmur versus pathological murmur by the primary care physician "more complex than is generally acknowledged" (McNamara, 1987b, p. 1161). These contributing factors to the diagnosis include a wide range of influences such as: What is the family's history concerning heart problems? (Goldfield et al., 1986); What is the physician's confidence in his or her training and expertise in the area of cardiology and has he or she maintained the skill by regular, if not daily, practice with patients? (Goldfield et al., 1986; McNamara, 1987a, 1987b); What type of tests and examinations are available to the physician upon which the diagnosis is to be made? (Hersher, 1988); and what are the time restraints/pressures of conducting the examination during a short office visit (McNamara, 1987a)?

In addition, physicians know they are "usually alerted to the presence of congenital heart disease or an acquired vascular heart disease by the discovery of a significant heart murmur" (Paraskos, 1988, p. 20). Therefore, the inappropriate diagnosis of an innocent heart murmur for a significant heart murmur can be life-threatening for the patient (Paraskos, 1988).

Another consideration for the primary care physician to weigh is the effect a referral to a pediatric cardiologist can have on the family and the patient in terms of stress and anxiety. Because of the seriousness of heart disease, the primary care physician may be reluctant to state definitely that the murmur is innocent. To be on the safe side, he or she may refer the patient to the heart specialist (Bergman & Stamm, 1967). But as Hersher (1988) contends, the act of such a referral implies that something could be seriously wrong with perhaps the most important organ in the body. Several recent articles (Hersher, 1988; McNamara, 1987b, 1988) address this very issue. How much anxiety and worry does the family experience when the child is referred for confirmation of an "innocent" murmur? While the physicians' position may be one of "little concern, but let's play it safe," the family's understanding may be more serious in nature. Indeed, how the doctor expresses the condition of the patient is often misunderstood by the family. For instance, one patient and family may not understand the difference between "heart disease" and "heart murmur" (Bergman & Stamm, 1967; Gidding & Rosenthal, 1984). A concern is that the family may continue to treat the child as being vulnerable to heart disease, surgery, or death (Green & Solnit, 1964) even after the diagnosis of benign murmur is upheld.

With all of this to consider, when an innocent heart murmur is detected, the primary care physician has at least three possible choices: (a) ignore the innocent murmur and say nothing to the parent; (b) tell the parent that the murmur is nothing serious, that it occurs in nearly half of all babies, and that it can be checked again at another time, or, in the instance of troublesome cases; (c) refer the patient to a pediatric cardiologist (McNamara, 1987b, 1988).

In summary, many writers who have concerned themselves with the referral process have proposed that referring physicians should weigh the potential harm of unnecessary worry against the potential danger of the ailment proving serious if the ailment is left unmentioned. Referral should be made, accordingly, only if the danger of a serious ailment outweighs the potential harm of unnecessary worry (Bergman & Stamm, 1967). But what should physicians say when they elect to refer a case? How should the referral be presented to the patient and/or family? The act of referral is not just a simple request on the part of the physician. It is also an act fraught with symbolism. No illness lacks its semantic dimension. The professional

> who feels involved exclusively in the maintenance of a physical mechanism and who dismisses the communicative aspects of this work operates on a simplistic and even dangerous premise. Human beings are not

> merely symbol users; every moment of their life is permeated with symbolism. (Barnlund, 1984, p. 42)

Charles Siebert (1990) specifically addresses the metaphorical nature of the heart in his article, *The Rehumanization of the Heart: What Doctors Have Forgotten, Poets Have Always Known*, and warns of possible dangers implicit in ignoring this view. He suggests that the consideration of the heart as only a pump to be treated by cardiac mechanics might lead to

> a subconscious rebellion against the demystification of the heart, the reduction of a once profound source of mystery and misgiving to a mere machine. In response to this medical reductionism, we may be suffering a kind of collective heart attack, a modern metaphysical one—pained by the weakening of long-held notions of the heart as the home of the soul and the seat of deep emotions. (p. 54)

There can be quite a contrast between how a physician understands a referral to a pediatric cardiologist and how a family interprets the same act, especially if the metaphoric nature of the heart is precluded. The doctor may frame the procedure as routine and unproblematic, but the family may choose to interpret the referral as being ominous and life-threatening. It is not clear from the literature that ways to address these differences in point of view, other than opting out of the referral process, are generally utilized and understood by physicians. In the instances when the physician is able to *identify* (Aylward, 1988) a suspected innocent heart murmur but is unable or unwilling to diagnose it as such and feels the need to refer the family to a pediatric cardiologist, how then can the referral be presented so that a minimal amount of worry and anxiety is aroused?

Aylward (1988) differentiated between identification and diagnosis of a problem. In regard to behavioral pediatrics, Aylward wrote, "Identification of a developmental problem may not be the same as diagnosis of the problem. . . . the pediatrician may suspect a problem and then refer the child to another professional such as a psychologist, speech pathologist, audiologist for confirmation" (p. 677). Confusion may arise because "in such circumstances, the parent may recall that the other professional made the diagnosis" (Aylward, 1988, p. 677).

In regard to heart murmurs, many physicians may not feel comfortable in diagnosing the nature of the murmur, but the doctors are still able to identify an irregularity in the child's heart. By definition, a murmur diagnosed as being innocent, is not a murmur that should bring great concern to parents, nor should the child have to be referred to a specialist. But in the case of a murmur being only identified, even when the innocent modifier is added, there is still a degree of uncertainty on the part of the physician and the parents, and there is still the need to have a pediatric cardiologist examine the child's heart. Identification needs confirmation, diagnosis does not.

In light of these concerns, certain questions arise: What does happen to a family once the doctor announces that the child has a heart murmur and that a referral is being made so that a pediatric cardiologist can further examine the child's heart? How do the parents derive meaning from this information? All of these queries indicate that a study of parents' concerns regarding their child's health should address meaning within a context (i.e., What happens to a family once they enter into a medical context that includes talk about a heart murmur?). One purpose of this report is to closely examine how families come to understand what it means to have a child with a heart murmur.

This researcher proposes that learning more about the process by which parents come to understand what a heart murmur means for them and their child consists of sitting down with the families, who have been referred to pediatric cardiologists, and simply asking them to give their impressions of: (a) how the heart murmur discovery occurred, (b) how the referral to the pediatric cardiologist was made, (c) what does having a child with a heart murmur mean to them, and (d) what their expectations for seeing a heart specialist are. The accounts, given by the parents, would provide an opportunity to draw distinctions so as to produce fine-grained descriptions of the parents' talk about the talk they have experienced since the discovery of the heart murmur.

A study of meaning from this perspective would hold that " 'meaning' may be regarded as an appropriate synonym of pattern, redundancy, information, and restraint" (Bateson, 1972, p. 130), and "any regularity discovered through research that describes a patterned and systematic association between two variables is itself context-dependent" (Mishler, 1979, p. 9). A study of parents' interpretations of the events surrounding their child's heart murmur, therefore, would entail describing the patterns of relationship between the parents' talk about the events of the referral, and the context in which these utterances were made. The context in this study could be the social domain (i.e., the medical system) in which the talk occurred, or the language in which the talk itself was embedded (e.g., how previous talk about the heart murmur creates a context for present talk regarding the murmur).

This process of meaning-construction is termed contextualization. Contextualization takes its meaning from the Latin roots: *com-*, which means together; plus *textere*, which means to join, to weave, or to plait.

The past participle of *contextere* is *contextus* which means coherence or sequence of words (*The American Heritage Dictionary of the English Language*, 1970, p. 288). From these roots, contextualization is taken to mean the process by which an individual joins or weaves words together such that coherence or meaning is produced. In the case of this research, the focus is on the ways parents contextualize or create coherence in their interactions with the medical system throughout the heart murmur discovery-referral process. At the same time, the parents' contextualizations are also understood as occurring within a context: The parents' talk about their child's heart is embedded within other types of talk (e.g., husband–wife relationship discussions), and social domains (e.g., familial, medical, cultural, etc.). A study of interactants' discourse must address not only the talk itself, but also the context in which the talk occurs, plus the relationship between the talk and its context.

Bateson (1979) wrote, "Without context, words and actions have no meaning at all. This is true not only of human communication in words but also of all communication whatsoever, of all mental process, of all mind" (p. 16). In some instances, the importance of studying contexts is taken for granted (for an expanded discussion see Mishler, 1979), but in this study, the focus is on what Bateson (1972) characterized as the evolving nature of "the qualitative structure of contexts" (p. 155).

Mishler (1979) added, "Human action can be understood only within its own context of socially grounded rules for defining, categorizing, and interpreting the meaning of our context" (p. 8). "The only way we can make sense of the world is to see the connections between things, and between present things and things we have experienced before or heard about. . . . As soon as we measure a new perception against what we know of the world from prior experience, we are dealing with expectations" (Tannen, 1979, p. 137). Tannen (1979) stated that these "structures of expectations" are sometimes called "schemas, scripts, or frames" (p. 138).

For the families to be interviewed, the questions would be: What are their expectations for seeing the cardiologist; how is the news of the heart murmur being framed; and what are the expectations for the child now that a heart murmur has been detected? These are the types of questions which concern many physicians and families (see Bergman & Stamm, 1967; Hersher, 1988; McNamara, 1988), but to this point in time have not been studied by any medical researchers in the way that has been suggested in this paper, although within the area of heart murmur/disease research itself there have been a few projects pertinent to the questions raised above.

PREVIOUS STUDIES

A search of medical literature reveals that there have been only a handful of studies which are relevant to this project: Glaser, Harrison, and Lynn's (1964) work with the emotional implications of congenital heart disease in children; Feinstein, Taube, Cavalieri, Schultz, and Kryle's (1962) examination of the relationship between physical activities and rheumatic heart disease in asymptomatic patients; Linde, Rasof, Dunn, and Rabb's (1966) research in attitudinal factors in congenital heart disease; Bergman and Stamm's (1967) study of the morbidity of cardiac nondisease in school children; and Park, Maddox, and Sridaromont's (1983) investigation of the psychological aspects of children with heart defects and their families.

The conclusions of all of these studies were best typified by Bergman and Stamm (1967, p. 1012) when they wrote, "The diagnosis of heart disease may cause profound changes in the functioning of a child and his [sic] family far beyond the immediate physical effects" Bergman and Stamm (1967, p. 1012), and the other researchers (see also Linde et al., 1966) based this conclusion on their observations that family members are less equipped than medical personnel to assess the degree of the severity, or nonseverity, of heart disease and/or heart murmurs. Because families can be confused over the seriousness/nonseriousness of a heart-related diagnosis, "too many people exist in an unnecessary limbo where they either perceive themselves or are perceived by others to have a nonexistent disease. Such a person may be disabled or 'unhealthy' as if he [sic] actually had the disease" (Bergman & Stamm, 1967, p. 1008).

The Bergman and Stamm (1967) paper was especially pertinent and informative to this investigation. In their study the two doctors surveyed 20,500 children in the Seattle public schools. Of these children, 110 parents reported that there was or had been " 'something' wrong with their child's heart" (p. 1009). Ninety-three of these children were given physicals and the parents were interested in ascertaining the relationship between the children's present medical conditions (i.e., the presence or absence of heart problems) and the treatments the children were receiving from their parents (i.e., the restrictions placed on the children's activities.

The results of the physical examinations revealed that 75 out of the 93 children, or 81 percent of "children whose parents reported to the schools that at one time 'something was wrong with the heart,' were found to have no present evidence of heart disease" (Bergman & Stamm, 1967, p. 1009), although 31 of the 75 or 42 percent of the children did have heart murmurs. Of the 75 children considered healthy by the physicians, 30 were judged to have been restricted by their parents in some way: The child was either treated as if handicapped in some way, restricted from some activities such as sports, or the parents expressed worry that something was wrong with the child (p. 1009).

Bergman and Stamm (1967) concluded that "the amount of disability from cardiac nondisease in children is estimated to be greater than due to actual heart disease" (p. 1013). In other words, that diagnoses, such as heart murmurs (a nondisease of the heart) can result in parents treating their children as if the children did indeed have heart disease.

When discussing reasons it would make sense for parents to restrict seemingly healthy children, Bergman and Stamm (1967) concluded that "the most decisive factor [for parents] whether or not a child was to be restricted appeared to be the advice of a physician" (p. 1013): 42 percent of the parents from the unrestricted group recalled that the physician had mentioned that the child would outgrow the condition and it should be ignored as compared to only 17 percent of the parents from the restricted group. Fifty-three percent of the parents from the restricted group recalled "receiving definite advice from the physician to curtail physical activities, versus 29% of the parents from the unrestricted group" (p. 1010).

For the parents in the restricted group, a context had been built in which treating their *healthy child* as an *unhealthy child* would make perfectly good sense. It was this reframing of the healthy child as unhealthy that served as the focus of the research: In what ways would the unhealthy-healthy child context be maintained, altered, or eliminated during the discovery and referral of a child for a heart murmur diagnosis?

Park (et al., 1983) at the Pediatric Cardiology Unit at Texas Tech University Health Sciences Center (TTUHSC) was also interested in studying how the discovery of heart murmurs and other heart nondiseases helped to shape parents' views of the children's health. In a project prior to the one discussed in this text, Park et al. (1983) had used surveys to ascertain family members' reactions to the discovery of a heart defect and/or a heart murmur in one of the children in the family. Park and his co-investigators had wanted to be able to study differences and similarities between the family members as to how the child with the heart murmur or heart defect was being contextualized. The results of the study were inconclusive, partially due to difficulties arising from methodological problems: The questionnaire developed for the project restricted the range of the parents' responses and, when parents were allowed to complete the forms at home, it was not certain whether or not two or one of the parents had filled out both of the questionnaires.

Park was still interested in studying the contextualizing effect of heart murmurs, when this author and his colleagues, Paul Douthit, Jerry Gale, and Jeff Stormberg, had an opportunity to develop a research program with Park and his colleagues, Drs. Somkid Sridaromont and Veronica Schmer (Park, Sridaromont, Schmer, Stormberg, Douthit, Gale, & Chenail, 1988), aimed at investigating family members' reactions to heart disease and/or murmur in their children. The immediate task faced by the group was to determine how family members could be assessed so as to better understand how the child was being contextualized. Dr. Park was especially interested in finding out how family members had constructed their views about the child between the time that the heart defect or murmur had been discovered and when the family made its initial visit to the pediatric cardiology unit at TTUHSC. The task of developing a way to understand this communication process was given to this author and his colleagues. The first step was to explore previous attempts of studying doctor–patient interactions and how these interactions helped to shape family members' understandings of health and disease.

COMMUNICATION IN MEDICINE AND THERAPY

A survey of the medical communication literature indicated that the general area is just beginning to be explored by sociologists, linguists, anthropologists, psychologists, and medical personnel (for general reviews see Cassata, 1978, 1980; Street, 1986; Street & Wiemann, 1987; Wasserman & Inui, 1983). One specialty of medical or health communication that was of special interest to this project was the study of doctor–patient interaction. Waitzkin (1984) stated that, although the literature on doctor–patient communication was fairly uninformative until the mid-1970s, in the past 15-plus years, "research in the social sciences has clarified the nature and the problems of doctor-patient communication" (p. 2441).

The exploration of this area of literature was guided by what Rogers (1987, p. 689) referred to when she discussed the fit between research and medical practice: What research approach on methodology would best fit with the problem at hand—the study of parents' interpretations of medical information regarding their child's heart condition?

> To improve fit: Ask questions, "What is the nature of the information about health and illness that we are generating? What models and meth-

> ods drive the work? . . . In a word, our aim is to assess social science research on health and illness for the purpose of suggesting how its findings may contribute to action strategies and relevance to health care. (Rogers, 1987, p. 689)

The logical question at that point was: What information was expected from this study and what means could be used to best produce and study this information? The doctors wanted to learn more about how parents and other family members were affected by the discovery of a heart murmur. In the previous study, (Park et al., 1983), survey methods had been used to assess familial attitudes. Two problems arose from using this approach: It was uncertain whether both parents were filling out the surveys, and, even if mothers and fathers both completed the form, would a quantitative analysis enable the doctors to examine how individuals were understanding the heart murmurs? The decision to consider alternatives to statistical means was supported by researchers, such as Rogers (1987), who wrote

> At the same time, we see in articles and books the limited explanatory power, for example, of contemporary quantitative research for understanding human behavior. Our corrective strategy tends to be: look for another model or measurement technique in the hope that we can thereby improve the variance explained. (p. 693)

Rather than study answers on a survey or questionnaire, it was decided that a more direct way to learn more about how parents understood their children's medical condition was to simply sit down with the families and talk with them about the circumstances at hand and then analyze the discourse to assess how parents were contextualizing their children's heart condition. This type of study would fall into the category of medical discourse: "face-to-face interaction between patients and practitioners in medical settings' (Freeman & Heller, 1987, p. 1). In the case of this study, the goals were to learn more about how family members came to construct the meaning of what was a heart murmur and how that construction affected the family's treatment of the child diagnosed as having the murmur To produce this type of information, discourse analysis of family interviews was chosen as the method by which to accomplish these goals.

Discourse analysis had been used to study a variety of medical, as well as therapeutic, phenomena (see Di Pietro, 1982; Fisher & Todd, 1983, 1986; Frankel, 1984b; Freeman & Heller, 1987) Discourse analysis had been employed in medicine to study: hedging in physician-physician discourse (Prince, Frader, & Bosk, 1982); miscommunication in physician-patient talk (West, 1984); negotiations over treatment between doctors and patients (Todd, 1984); how different contexts shape medical communication (Tannen & Wallat, 1986); and basic descriptions of the medical interview (Frankel, 1984a; Worobey, O'Hair, & O'Hair, 1987; Raimbault, Cachin, Limal, Eliacheff, & Rappaport, 1975). In therapy, discourse analysis has been utilized to describe: the relationship between language patterns and therapeutic change (Labov & Fanshel, 1977; Phoenix & Lindeman, 1982); restructuring intervention in family therapy (Troemel-Ploetz, 1977); problem presentation in therapy and interviews (Wodak, 1981); "problem (re)formulation" in therapy (Davis, 1986, p. 44); blaming and accounting in couples therapy (Buttny, in press); and framing problems in therapy (Buttny & Lannamann, 1986).

Although some interesting results have been produced through the use of discourse analysis in medical and therapeutic settings (see Shuy, 1984, for a review), many researchers contended that much more needed to be accomplished. Rogers (1987) warned "to learn more about social behavior and its influences, we need process data, yet relatively little work has been undertaken in this direction" (p. 693). This position was also supported by Freeman (1987), who wrote that the study of communication in the medical setting was "in a continuing need for basic descriptive work" and "still in the process of developing an understanding of the dimensions of routine medical interaction of various kinds" (p. 3). Wasserman and Inui (1983) also concurred by stating that "surprisingly little is known about the interaction, their antecedents, and their effects" (p. 279).

Because so little was known about how meaning was constructed in face-to-face interaction in medical settings, the investigation of the interviews would be conducted along discovery-oriented lines (e.g., Hopper, 1988; Mahrer, 1988). The purpose of the discovery-oriented approach, as compared to an experimental one, would be to learn more about the basic interactions rather than to set about confirming or disconfirming hypotheses. There did not seem to be enough theory surrounding doctor-patient interaction so as to construct hypotheses to support an experimental design. This study was seen as a way to contribute data that could possibly lead to later, experimental studies (see further discussion in Chapter 5).

MEANING AND CONTEXT

After perusing the literature, it became clear that one possible reason why such a study, as proposed in this chapter, has not been undertaken is how the relationship between meaning and context is usually approached in theory and research.

> One side of the paradox is that we all know that human action and experience are context dependent and can only be understood within their contexts. . . . The other side of the paradox is that this ordinary and commonsense understanding of meaning as context dependent has been excluded from the main tradition of theory and research in the social and psychological sciences. . . . As theorists and researchers, we tend to behave as if context were the enemy of understanding rather than the resource for understanding which it is in our everyday life. (Mishler, 1979, p. 2)

In order for questions, like the ones raised above, to be answerable, different approaches and metaphors have to be found so that meaning within context can be studied in a medical or any of a variety of settings. Mishler (1979) suggested "a number of alternative approaches and methods may be more appropriate including methods drawn from ecological psychology, phenomenology research, sociolinguistics, and ethnomethodology" (p. 17). All of these approaches consider the study of meaning within a context to be a resource, rather than something for which controls must be designed so as to insure the validity of the results.

Another approach, which also has been applied to the study of communication and behavior within a context, is systemic family therapy (see Keeney, 1983). This type of family therapy, sometimes also known as systems therapy or systemic therapy, refers to those clinicians/researchers who apply systems principles in their work (Simon, Stierlin, & Wynne, 1985). Three major distinctions that have been used to organize systemic family therapy are "(1) a problem-solution interactional focus; (2) a triadic social relations focus; and (3) a contextual meaning focus" (Keeney & Ross, 1985, p. 5).

For the purposes of this study, taking a systemic family perspective means that an emphasis is placed on understanding how the words and actions of the parents, in regard to their child's heart murmur and their involvement with the medical system, make sense within a context. In other words, how does it make sense for parents to treat their child, who has an innocent heart murmur, as if the child had heart disease? By attending to how the parents, through interaction with each other, the doctors, and other involved parties (e.g., grandparents, friends, and neighbors), have constructed a context in which a heart murmur becomes synonymous with heart disease, a systemic family therapy researcher can make an important contribution to medicine's understanding of what can happen to families when a heart murmur is discovered.

Besides providing descriptions of the family members' interpretations, another purpose of this study is to present a variety of prescriptions to participants in the heart murmur discovery/referral process. These prescriptions, based on distinctions drawn in the descriptions of the family members' talk about their experiences, are intended to help physicians and parents alike, to organize and to manage information. By doing so, the meaning of the heart murmur and the significance of the referral to a pediatric cardiologist can be contextualized in a less worrisome manner than was experienced by some families in the study.

Again, a systemic family therapist perspective is advantageous to this endeavor. Systemic family therapists understand that their descriptions of the families shape what is prescribed for those families, and, at the same time, the prescriptions will also help to form and reform the therapists' view of the family. Whether that prescription is a behavioral intervention or a reframing of the families' understanding of the situation at hand, the therapist's descriptions contextualize the prescriptions and vice versa.

The descriptions provided in this text may be taken as prescriptions for how participants in the heart murmur discovery-referral process could organize information such that worry and concern could be minimized. In addition, based upon the descriptions provided, doctors and family members may be able to create their own prescriptions for handling interactions during their encounters.

Considerable support for involving a systemic view in medicine is readily found in both the family therapy and medical literature. A family and/or systems approach has already been incorporated in many areas of medical treatment and understanding, such as: with diabetes (Caldwell & Pichert, 1985); with family medicine (Doherty & Baird, 1983, 1987; Glenn, 1985; Schwartzman, 1985); with pediatrics (Montalvo, Schor, & Moore, 1987; Sargent, 1985); with total health care (Rinaldi, 1985); with rehabilitation (Peck, 1974); and with compliance (Stein & Pontious, 1985).

To study heart murmur referrals to pediatric cardiologists from a systems perspective seems especially relevant given that "pediatrics is inherently a family focused specialty" (Munson, 1986, p. 234). In pediatrics, and also with family medicine, the unit of treatment is often the family (Doherty & Baird, 1983), and systemic family therapists can contribute to the care of these patients and their families. One way in which therapists can complement physicians who utilize a family perspective in their treatment of patients is to act as consultants in the proceedings. Consultation of this sort could be heavily oriented towards offering the staff a treatment plan to deal with the family and also to broaden the staff's understandings of (a) the stressor currently experienced by the family; (b) the family interaction pattern; (c) how and what the family is able to communicate, especially about the illness; and (d) how the staff affects the family (Wellisch & Cohen, 1986, p. 200).

It may seem obvious that physicians should consider these issues, but "specific transactional problems between the families and staff members are worthy of special note because of their relative frequency and the ease with which they are overlooked" (Munson, 1986, p. 234).

> It is appropriate as well to consider the meaning of these events for the family system. . . it is well to recognize that the disease, or treatment, or the relationship with the health care providers is significantly meaningful to the family system. (Bloch, 1986, p. 146)

Besides helping physicians to understand treatment from a systemic perspective, family therapists can also lend aid by consulting when specific problems arise when dealing with families. Therapists could contribute in "the development of strategies for managing issues arising from the interlocking triangles of the patient family, the provider family, and the treatment system" (McDaniel, Bank, Campbell, Mancini, & Shore, 1986, p. 196). The descriptions and prescriptions outlined in this study help to continue the productive collaboration between family therapists and physicians: Given the difficulties that can arise during the discovery/referral sequence, therapists-as-consultants can prove to be valuable resources for primary care physicians and specialists alike, in helping families through a difficult process.

In contrast to the abundance of examples citing the contributions of family therapy to treatment, there are only a few instances of family or systemic perspectives being incorporated into medical research (e.g., Anderson & Kornblum, 1984; Tannen & Wallat, 1983, 1986). "The family therapist rarely serves as consultant to biomedical research enterprises. This is unfortunate because a substantial contribution ought to be forthcoming in this direction, particularly in regards to the inclusion of the family systems variable" (Bloch, 1986, p. 145). This research project serves as a major step in bridging the gap between medical and systemic family therapy research by demonstrating that significant findings can be accomplished through the cooperative efforts of systemic family therapy and pediatric medicine.

This bridging of a gap between systemic or family therapy and medical research finds support in a considerable body of literature which advocates an expanded relationship between medical and social science research in general (see Rogers, 1987). These recommendations range from Banta's (1983) position that "the development and implementation of public policy towards medical technology would profit if social science were to become involved in its examination" (p. 1363); to Hull's (1987) statement that

> a most important role of socio-behavioral scientists lies in helping the medical profession to remove the attitudinal and educational barriers which prevent the realisation of the concept of a new sort of doctor who may cope with the demands of primary health care as we approach 2000. (p. 679)

Waitzkin (1984) went further in making a case for the incorporating social science research into the study of medicine by citing some of the progress brought about past interdisciplinary endeavors:

> Research in the social sciences has clarified the nature and the problems of doctor-patient communication. The development of adequate communication skills is now the goal of training in the primary care specialties. (p. 2441)

Social science research has already had an influence in medical practice, and now systemic family therapy, too, has an opportunity to contribute to this process, the benefits of which could also be felt in the research conducted in our own field.

> Our goal is to improve the fit between social science and health practice by increasing the relevance of social science findings for the delivery of care and the training of health care professionals. In addition, hopefully, our suggestions will advance social science research independent of its impact on the health care. (Rogers, 1987, p. 689)

Although interdisciplinary research between social science and medicine is not without its critics (see Niklas, 1982), there seem to be some definite advantages to the introduction of systemic family therapy ideas into medical research. This study demonstrates that a project involving family therapy and medical perspectives can prove fruitful to both disciplines in terms of a cross-fertilization of ideas and methods. In addition, the findings of this project could prove beneficial to patients, parents, physicians, and therapists involved in the health care system.

Chapter 2 concentrates on (a) demonstrating the utility of approaching the study of this influence from a communication perspective; (b) establishing the credibility of employing discourse analysis as a means to understand and describe families' experiences as they attempt to make sense of their interactions while being in the medical system; and (c) outlining the origins and development of the type of discourse analysis employed in this study, Recursive Frame Analysis (RFA), and arguing the relevance of RFA as method of choice in this study. Chapter 2 concludes with a discussion of how this project specifically addresses the study of the heart murmur discovery/referral process.

Chapter 3 demonstrates the methodology employed in this study. Included in this chapter is a discussion on the selection of families interviewed for the project, on the procedures followed in recording and transcribing the interviews, and on the analysis employed in the examination of the family members' discourse concerning their experiences during the discovery/referral sequence.

Chapter 4 presents the detailed analysis of the excerpts drawn from the families' interviews. Recursive Frame Analysis (Keeney, 1990a, 1990b) is utilized to draw basic distinctions to understand how families organized their experiences surrounding the referral to a pediatric cardiologist, and how the family members contextualized the meaning of the heart murmur.

Chapter 5 takes the descriptions, detailed in Chapter 4, and uses these to suggest ways in which participants in the heart murmur discovery/referral process can organize and manage information and contexts. The prescriptions are suggested so as to help doctors and family members in their interactions with each other during the difficult, somewhat confusing, sometime worrisome, referral sequence. The chapter concludes with a discussion on ways to disseminate the findings of this study, and also on how this project informs subsequent studies.

The examination of families' interpretations of their experiences with their children's heart murmurs is guided by the words of George Miller (as cited in Lakoff & Ross, 1979, p. viii): "In order to understand what another person is saying, you must assume it is true and try to imagine what it could be true of." It is not the purpose of this investigation to question family's realities in light of a true, real world, but rather, to try to understand each family member's own unique logic and vision; and how presenting descriptions of these individualized distinctions can be helpful to other families and physicians who must also deal with this aspect of the human condition.

Chapter 2
The Study of Talk and Recursive Frame Analysis

INTRODUCTION

In Chapter 1 the general area to be investigated was established: The research would focus on how family members were informed of the news that one of the children in the family was diagnosed as having a heart murmur. Background material in the biological nature of murmurs was presented, as well as some of the concerns that doctors and researchers had in regards to the influences that the heart murmur discovery and subsequent referral to a pediatric cardiologist had on family members' perceptions of the child with the murmur.

The survey continued by examining the previous studies in which researchers and physicians attempted to study the family interaction surrounding the heart murmur discovery. The section concluded with a summary that highlighted the important findings and features of these studies.

In Chapter 2, the center of attention is talk and the ways in which discourse can be understood and studied. In the previous chapter the argument was made for studying language in the field of medicine. In this chapter, the discussion picks up at that point and the reader is introduced to a mode of inquiry which allows investigators to focus on such phenomena. Methods used in previous medical and therapy studies are critiqued and other alternative means used to study language and discourse, such as narrative analysis, are introduced so as to improve the fit between the information to be studied and the methods to be used in this study. The utility of frames and frame analysis in the analysis of discourse and narrative will be emphasized in this section and a new method for studying and understanding talk will be introduced: Recursive Frame Analysis (RFA).

Chapter 2 concludes with a focused presentation of the problem to be studied. The important distinctions that organize the methodological choices taken and the scope of the analysis will also be discussed.

DISCOURSE ANALYSIS

The literature did supply a general orientation to the study of doctor-patient interaction, which helped to shape the context for this study. Especially important in this orientation process was the role language played in medicine.

> The day-to-day practice of medicine is built upon verbal exchanges, making events susceptible to linguistic analysis, and as Mishler points out, "In this approach, the grounds for interpretation are located in the perspective of patients and the life world contexts of their problems rather than in the biomedical perspective of physician." (Shuy, 1984, p. 422)

Linguists, like Shuy, strongly advocated that physicians, besides analyzing test results, should also become aware of the patients' view of the medical situation. Waitzkin (1985) has also noted that

> Doctors and patients frequently frame their communication on the basis of their unspoken perceptions concerning each other's expectations in the situation. In framing their remarks, doctors may make benign judgments about what patients want to know or should know, but the basis of such judgments may be problematic. (p. 2442)

One empirical way to evaluate patients' perspectives was to carefully analyze the speech of patients. The study of patients' language enabled researchers to show "that patients came prepared with some idea to what is wrong, whilst other patients seem less prepared, but equally in need of information as well as advice and treatment" (Wadsworth, 1976, p. 6).

The formal study of patients' talk would fall under the general rubric of discourse analysis. This type of analysis focuses on "that level of linguistic analysis which considers any linguistic unit larger than the sentence, whether it is a unit of interactional structure, . . . , or a unit of linguistic structure, the discourse unit" (Linde, 1986, p. 184). The study of discourse was emphasized in the study of doctor-patient talk because "discourse is the linguistic level at which social action and exchange takes place. That is, we do not exchange sentences or words or such" (Linde, 1986, p. 184). Although some critics (see Frawley, 1987a) argued that formal grammar was capable of studying units larger than a sentence, a majority of discourse analysts have decided that, rather than analyze talk from a grammar perspective of sentence and paragraph, instead, they have chosen to use discourse units such as "the narrative, small group planning, explanation, description, argument, command and control discourse in commercial aviation, etc." (Linde, 1986, p. 184) as distinctions to be studied in talk.

In addition, Linde (1986, p. 184) also stressed that the discourse unit be studied "as part of the wider context in which it is embedded." From this perspective, the researcher, as well as the doctor and patient, needed to pay special attention to context. Agar (1985, p. 148) called this view of discourse analysis "context type," wherein the investigator attempted to "represent an intermediate level between the human contact that led to the discourse and the broader characteristics of the society in which it is embedded." From Agar's perspective, a map constructed by investigators to study doctor-patient interaction should chart the verbal exchanges and at the same time, acknowledge the social context in which the talk was being spoken.

"The physician learns that he or she is always working within a complex interlacing of contexts" (Stein & Pontious, 1985, p. 189): The talk between the physician and the patient is embedded within a larger body of discourse which is the social context of the talk, and within the doctor–patient interaction itself, the words of the participants become embedded within other words and this is also understood as context. "And 'context' is linked to another undefined notion called 'meaning.' Without context, words and actions have no meaning at all. This is true not only of human communication in words but also of all communication whatsoever, of all mental process, of all mind" (Bateson, 1979, p. 16). Surprisingly, many researchers ignore the interactional qualities of interaction. Street (1986) wrote "researchers generally do not consider such as the participants' response contingencies, how interactants coordinate mutual or competing goals and expectancies, how behavioral patterns evolve during the course of interaction, and what cognitive affective factors influence these processes" (p. 227).

One way to assess these cognitive affective factors or *schemas* (Tannen & Wallat, 1986, p. 299) which influence interaction would be to examine closely surface evidence for these underlying expectancies. The study of the relationship between these psychological schemas and observable interactions was first outlined by Bateson (1979) in his study of *frames* (see Coyne, 1985; Goffman, 1974; Keeney, 1990b; Tannen, 1979).

FRAMES

Bateson introduced the notion of frame during his discussions on play (Bateson, 1956, 1972). He was interested in discerning how animals and people were able to differentiate between what was play and what was not play. When was a bite all in play, and when did the nip become the first step towards a fight? Bateson believed that participants had the ability to metacommunicate about their communication so that, during interaction, they would be able to give each other messages, such as *This is play*, so that each would understand how the behavior or communication should be understood. Bateson said that messages like *This is play* helped to establish a frame or context for the biting communication (Bateson, 1972, pp. 178–184).

Bateson (1972, p. 186) considered frame and context to be psychological concepts and he used the analogies of a picture frame and mathematical set theory to discuss these ideas. He said that a picture frame gave an indication that the contents of that frame should be considered differently than other objects on the wall, such as the wallpaper. A mathematical set theory formed rules which "set membership and nonmembership" for that set. Bateson (1972) defined a psychological frame by stating that "it is (or delimits) a class or set of messages (or meaningful actions)" (p. 186).

Bateson (1972, pp. 187–188) outlined seven functions and uses of psychological frames. Among these functions were the notions of exclusivity and inclusivity, the metacommunicative nature of frames, and the embeddedness of frames. As was the case of a mathematical set theory, exclusivity of a frame meant frames dictated what would not belong within that context, and inclusivity of a frame meant that frames also dictated what would belong within that context. Frames were metacommunicative because they were attempts to define the meaning of messages, and, conversely, every metacommunicative message also was or defined a frame. Finally, frames were understood as being embedded because frames were also understood within contexts: The frame of a frame gave the receiver messages about the meaning of the included frame.

Bateson (1972, p. 187) believed that an onlooker could observe outward signs of these psychological frames. These signs were to be found in participants' language and behaviors. "We assume that the psychological frame has some degree of real existence. In many instances, the frame is consciously recognized and even represented in vocabulary ("play," "movie," "interview," "job," "language," etc.). In other cases, there may be no explicit verbal reference to the frame, and the subject may have no consciousness of it" (Bateson, 1972, pp. 186–187).

The influence of psychological frames on verbalizations were not taken to be unidirectional nor was the relationship seen to be rigid in nature:

> The fluidity and lability of frames, however, derived from the reflexive nature of messages which simultaneously constituted and labeled them. Consider: when was a shove too hard or a remark too hurtful to maintain a perception of the interaction as play? What behavioral "cues" certified our perceptions? (Rawlins, 1987, p. 58)

This mutual shaping process between the frame and that which was framed was expressed in the title of Bateson's (1956) talk at one of the Macy Conferences: "The message 'This is play' " (p. 145).

> The frame itself thus became part of the premise system. Either, as in the case of the play frame, the frame was involved in the evaluation of the message which it contained, or the frame merely assisted the mind in understanding the contained messages by reminding the thinker that these messages were mutually relevant and the message outside the frame was ignored. (Bateson, 1979, p. 188)

The understanding or framing of what play was was constructed by comparing behavior that was contextualized as being play with the play frame itself. There was always a degree of flexibility within a frame.

> A child realized that behavior can, in a sense, be set to a logical type or to a style. It was not the learning of the particular style that you were playing at, but the fact of stylistic flexibility and the fact that the choice of style or role was related to the frame and context of the behavior. And play itself was a category of behavior, classified by context in some way. (Bateson, 1956, pp. 148–149)

Alton Becker (1984a) was also interested in how context and language interacted: "In what ways context constrains particular language—real text (i.e., remembered or preserved language). There are many ways to answer that question, depending on how one defines context. One way to see context is as sources of constraints on text" (p. 136).

Becker stated that such constraints consisted of the relation between prior and current talk (i.e., how previous talk about the child's heart murmur constrained current talk about the child); the relation between the talk and the participants creating said talk (i.e., how talk between a parent and a doctor over a child's heart murmur might differ from talk between two parents about their child's heart murmur); and the relation between the talk and the medium in which that talk was delivered (i.e., how parents' talk about their child's heart murmur during a visit with a nurse might differ from parents' talk about the murmur with a pediatric cardiologist). The interaction of all of these restraints helped to shape the talk, and, at the same time, the talk helped to reshape its own context.

Although there is a degree of flexibility and reflexivity between the interaction of constraints on text, problems can arise when a degree of rigidity is introduced within the system. When referring to a schizophrenic patient with whom he had been playing golf, Bateson (1956) said, "I am concerned how to illustrate how play sets a frame for behavior. There was a frame set for a certain style of action, and within this frame he could function. But when the frame was modified by competition and when he started to fail it became a little harder" (p. 149). In this instance Bateson could have been talking about "competition" as a frame which contextualized another frame "play," or competition could have referred to an observable interaction which helped to reshape the frame of play. In turn, the behavior became to be understood within a new and different context (competition). This behavior/frame interaction was what Bateson (1956) referred to when he stated, "I am speaking especially of those messages which define context; the message, 'This is play,' which I have taken as text, is a message defining context in a way, or defining a frame" (p. 163).

Goffman (1974) also expressed his concern about frame reification when he wrote

> Activities . . . tend to foreclose other frame possibilities and require sustaining a definition of the situation in the face of diversions. Once initiated, these activities must find a place in the ongoing world, and the ongoing world must find a palpable place for them. (p. 499)

In the case of parents with a child who has been diagnosed as having a heart murmur, the message, *This is heart murmur*, can help the family come to understand that their child is an unhealthy child. If the frame of unhealthy child becomes rigid in its application, there will be a lack of flexibility in the treatment of that child. This was seen in the Bergman and Stamm (1967) study: The style of parent-child interaction for some of the families had become stuck in a vulnerable/unhealthy child framework. Just as the schizophrenic man described by Bateson above had trouble accepting that golf as play can also be golf as competition, some families, who understood that their child had a heart murmur, had trouble understanding that their child was also healthy. The understanding of the diagnosis of an innocent heart murmur as meaning unhealthy child, and the behavior associated with that logic, was the focus of this study.

NARRATIVE ANALYSIS

This project was part of a larger research project which had as its goal the investigation of the communication process which began with a hearing of the frames introduced to the parents in the referring physician's office, which continued with an examination of the frames negotiated in the pediatric cardiologist's office, and which concluded with a testing of the resiliency of frames in a follow-up visit with the family. The data for the project came from interviews with parents who had been referred to see a pediatric cardiologist because of their child's heart condition. Just prior to their seeing the pediatric cardiologist at the hospital, parents were given an opportunity to present what Webb and Stimson (1976, p. 108) called "lay accounts." The interview would be a way to take a sample from a process which started with

> the person's consultation with a general practitioner as part of an extended process involving the patient-to-be [and parents] in a whole series of prior anticipations, expectations, and preparations for the encounter, and, after the consultation was over, involving the person in evaluation and appraisal. It would be during this time and reappraisal and evaluation when there would be verbal accounts of "what really happened." (Webb & Stimson, 1976, p. 108)

The interview would be a way to find out "what really happened," or rather, how the family members made sense of the past events (i.e., the discovery, diagnosis, and referral events). The story presented by the parents would not be used for a comparative study to measure what was recalled by the parents with what was reported by the physician (see Kosa, Albert, & Haggerty, 1967). Following Webb and Stimson (1967), the purpose of this analysis was

> not to make any claims about the correspondence between what was depicted in the stories and what "independent observers" might have agreed to what had happened at the incident in question. The interest was in the way the stories were told and not in questions of the validity of the accounts. (p. 110)

Webb and Stimson (1967, p. 122) "chose to use the term 'account' to describe the process of describing these events, rather than a term such as 'recall' which capitalized on notions of validity." This position was similar to the one espoused by Goffman (1974): "A replaying, in brief, recounts a personal experience, not merely reports on an event" (p. 504).

Analysis of these stories or accounts would fall under a specialization of discourse analysis referred to as *narrative analysis* (Gulich & Quasthoff, 1986a, 1986b; Linde, 1986; Wiedemann, 1986; Wodak, 1986). A narrative would be considered "a type of discourse unit" (Linde, 1986, p. 184) in which the talk or text "must recapitulate events from the past" (Gulich & Quasthoff, 1986b, p. 219). In nontechnical terms, a narrative can be an oral or written story in which past happenings are retold to a listening or reading audience. According to Gulich and Quasthoff (1986b), an analysis of a narrative could include *sequential analysis* and/or *semantic analysis* (p. 232) of the story-telling.

> Besides the precise nature of the narrative account, the investigator would also be very much concerned with the problem of what data needed to be made explicit for an analysis to be made: such matters as the situation in which the narration took place, the conversational context, the relationship between the narrator and his [sic] audience, etc. (Gulich & Quasthoff, 1986b, p. 220)

Gulich's, Quasthoff's, and the other narrative analysts' recommendations for the study of narratives were reminiscent of Becker's constraints that were discussed above: To understand the meaning of a story, the contexts within and without must be examined. This was similar to Bateson's (1979) notion of story, "I have suggested that it [story] had something to do with context, a crucial concept, partly undefined and therefore to be examined" (p. 16).

The parents' story was also seen as being a context. The story of the child's heart murmur helped to shape the family members' understanding of the child's condition (i.e., healthy or unhealthy). By hearing the parents' accounts of their interaction with the medical system during the discovery and referral for their child's heart murmur, an investigator or physician could begin to have an idea of what the heart murmur meant to the family and how this meaning was framing the parents' views of the child.

Another factor to consider in the study of the family members' stories was how should the structural and/or semantic analysis of the narrative be conducted? Declaring that this study was a narrative analysis only constrained the unit of analysis, and did not necessarily dictate the means for analyzing the meaning and structure of the accounts. Conversational analysis, ethnomethodology, and pragmatics were just a few of a variety of approaches used in previous studies of narratives (see Gulich & Quasthoff, 1986a), but for this study another method was chosen to provide a way to describe the organization of the discourse (sequential analysis), as well as to illustrate the embedded contexts of the talk (semantic analysis). The method of analysis chosen for this study was Recursive Frame Analysis (RFA), a method developed by Bradford Keeney (1990a, 1990b) and built upon the notions of frame: as a way of indicating the name of a context and as a way of visualizing the organization of conversations (1990a, p. 40).

RECURSIVE FRAME ANALYSIS

The notion of frames, as applied through the utilization of frame analysis, had been used to study a variety of topics: family dysfunction (Ariel, 1987); doctor-patient discourse (Evans, Block, Steinberg, & Penrose, 1986); general human interaction ranging from con games to professional wrestling and from literature to television (Goffman, 1974); family violence (Keeney & Bobele, 1989); and expectations about events and objects (Tannen, 1979). All of the studies varied in the way in which the idea of frames was applied to the subject matter. One variation that was commonly seen was the way in which the researchers conceptualized the rigidity in the relationship between the frame and that which was framed. In other words, some studies portrayed the frame/content relationship as being static: A frame framed the content in a narrow sense—there was not a sense of reciprocity between the content and its frame (Ariel, 1987). Other studies (i.e., Goffman, 1974) suggested that the researcher take an *as if* stance on the relationship between the frame and the content of that frame: Analyze the interaction as if the relationship between the frame and the framed was unidirectional and then see what picture is produced from the analysis of the speakers' interaction.

However tortured the connection can become between last person's talk and current speaker's utterances, that connection must be explored under the auspices of determinism, as though all the degrees of freedom available to whosoever is about to talk can somehow be mapped out, conceptualized, and ordered, somehow neatly grasped and held, somehow made to submit to the patterning-out effected by the analysis. If contents can be grouped into categories according to the ways in which they render the standard force of an utterance inapplicable and principles thus developed for determining when this meaning will be set aside, then such must be attempted. Similarly, sequencing must be anticipated and described (Goffman, 1981, p. 72).

In his analysis of human interaction, Goffman (1974) focused on the relationship between "inner thoughts" and "outer speech" (p. 503) as he studied the "the analysis of the strips of activity," with special emphasis on "the analysis of the act of saying things" (p. 496). Outer speech or utterances were understood as being "anchored in the surrounding, ongoing world" (p. 500). His view of frame analysis attempted to examine "the shape and character of these vehicles [utterances] which carry our burden": the ordeal of expressing inner thoughts through words (p. 503).

Tannen (1979) approached the subject from a perspective that was less deterministic than Goffman's, but she was also interested in examining the relationship of frames, or as she referred to them—expectancies, to subsequent events.

> The only way we can make sense of the world is to see the connection between things, and between present things and things we have experienced before or heard about. . . . As soon as we measure a new perception against what we know of the world from prior experiences, we are dealing with expectations. (p. 137)

In her version of frame analysis, Tannen (1979) wanted "to illustrate a way of showing the effects of those "structures of expectations" or verbalizations in the telling of oral narratives" (p. 138). Yet, the emphasis in her analysis seemed to focus on a one-way relationship between the frame and what it framed.

Keeney (1983, 1987a, 1987b, 1990a, 1990b), in contrast to Goffman and Tannen, presented a variation on the notion of frames and frame analysis. He stressed that frames were always understood as being embedded within other frames and each frame contextualized and, in turn, was contextualized by another frame (Keeney, 1987b). This in itself was not unique as far as frames had been presented before.

Goffman (1974) had written about embeddedness when he described the notion of *lamination* (p. 82). For Goffman, the initial framing of an utterance was termed the *primary framework*: the first context in which the talk was understood (p. 82). As time and interaction continued, additional frames, or *keyings* as he called them, contextualized the original frame/content relationship, and the meaning was transformed (p. 82). Goffman wrote, "It became convenient to think of each transformation as adding a layer of lamination to the activity" (p. 82). Also, the "keyings themselves were subject to rekeying" and the process of meaning became "a transformation of transformations" (p. 156), until what the observer observed or, rather, constructed were "multiple laminations of experience" (p. 182).

What did make Keeney's (1990a, 1990b) view and application of frames different from previous attempts such as Tannen's and Goffman's was Keeney's notion of form (Keeney, 1983; Spencer-Brown,

1972) and recursion (Keeney, 1983; von Foerster, 1984a, 1984b). The incorporation of these two concepts into his understanding made Keeney's presentation of frames different from previous utilizations.

Keeney's frame analysis was influenced by the work of G. Spencer-Brown (1972) on the mathematics of form (see Keeney, 1987b). The naming of a frame, or as Spencer-Brown (1972) called the process—the drawing of a distinction (p. 1), meant that an observer drew a distinction such that "a universe would come into being when a space was severed or taken apart" (p. xxix). This universe was made up of that which was named (the frame), and that which was not named (i.e., "that and that from which it was defined," p. 4). "Once a distinction was drawn, the spaces, states, or contents on each side of the boundary, being distinct, could be indicated" (p. 1). A frame was understood only in relation to what it framed.

Keeney's idea of frame contrasted with those theorists who presented a deterministic picture of frames (i.e., a frame determined the context of an utterance.) Bateson (1972, p. 155) discussed that at one time, he also made the error of thinking that context had unilateral control over content, but later, he clearly outlined how he came to understand context.

> I speak of an action or utterance as occurring "in" a context, and this conventional way of talking suggests that the particular action is a "dependent" variable, which the context is the "independent" or determining variable. But this view of how an action is related to its context is likely to distract the reader—as it has distracted me—from perceiving the ecology of the ideas which constitute the small subsystem which I call "context."
>
> It is important to see the particular utterance or action as *part* [emphasis from the original source] of the ecological subsystem called context and not as the product or effect of what remains of the context after the piece which we want to explain has been cut out from it. (Bateson, 1972, p. 338)

Keeney's understanding of frame, as influenced by Bateson, (i.e., the frame itself, that which was framed, and the relationship between the two sides of the distinction) evoked a pattern similar to what Spencer-Brown (1972) referred to as form: "Call the space cloven by any distinction, together with the entire context of the space, the form of the distinction" (p. 4). The act of framing was a choice of an observer as to how a sequence may be punctuated or understood. The understanding was not that a frame determined the meaning of what was framed, but rather, both the frame and what was framed were understood by the relationship drawn by the observer.

As was the case with Goffman's (1974) transformations of transformations, the forming of forms was an ongoing process. Keeney (1983) characterized this process as being recursive in nature.

> Cybernetics, circularity, repetition, recurrence, redundancy, pattern—all refer to recursion. These terms suggest that the ideas, experience, and social events do more than stretch out in lineal time. When a process infolds upon itself, we speak of recursion. The image of a circle is probably not the best way to think of recursion since we are not really referring to a return to an original beginning point in time. Each recursive loop does imply a different beginning, although in terms of the pattern of organization, it is simply recycled. (Keeney, 1983, pp. 582–59)

Although observers may punctuate in terms of hierarchy "we should not forget that this hierarchy is recursively structured" (Keeney, 1983, p. 31). For frames and frame analysis, this meant that the form of the frame folded back upon itself each time the form was evoked by an observer. This did not necessarily mean that each new cycle determined a new meaning for the frame, but rather that each recursive cycle created the possibility of a new combination or pattern to emerge, and each new pattern would be based upon the same rules of form under which the first distinction drawing was understood. This was similar to the point von Foerster (1984b) made when he wrote, "the recursive operation is a principle of self-organization . . . allowed certain structures to emerge—to crystalize—from early, arbitrary stages" (p. 19).

For some (see Wynne, 1988; Greenberg, 1989), the idea of recursion suggested a unidirectional flow of causality, and thus was just another way to continue with a linear/lineal view of cause and effect. This was the same error Bateson (as cited in Keeney, 1983) was referring to when he wrote

> [My colleagues in the behavioral sciences] have tried to build a bridge to the wrong half of the ancient dichotomy between form and substance. The conservative laws for energy and matter concern substance rather than form. But mental process, ideas, communication, organization, differentiation, pattern, and so on, are matters of form and substance. (p. 80)

From this discussion, it can be seen that recursion was used to name a pattern of context that had emerged over time, and not as a way to describe a circular version of unidirectional control.

Seymour Papert (1980), one of the founders of the computer language *Logo*, supplied a recursion riddle which helped to explain the difference between recursion as a directional concept and recursion as a meaning concept. Papert wrote: "If you have two wishes, what is the second? (Two more wishes)" (p. 74). The phrase, "two more wishes," was an answer in the context of the question "If you have two wishes, what is the second?" The question did not cause the answer, rather the phrase took on the meaning of an answer within the context of a question/answer relationship or form.

The unfolding of the process upon itself (i.e., the opportunity to receive two more wishes and to ask for two more wishes) was not caused by the wish of two wishes nor by the asking of the question regarding the nature of a second wish. The humor, the childlike quality, of the riddle and the recursiveness of the process suggested by the words come from the form of the riddle (i.e., the question, the answer, and the relationship between the two sides of the distinction), and not from any uni-, bi-, or multidirectionality of the phrases. The notions of context and directionality suggested two different epistemologies: one of pattern (context) and one of cause and effect (directionality).

William Gephart's (1981) description of watercolor painting served as another metaphor to understand recursion as a process of meaning or framing:

> For example, when a brush loaded with water and pigment is applied to a sheet of watercolor it will leave on the paper a brilliant area of the color deposited by that pigment. Ten to fifteen minutes later the water deposited with that pigment will have evaporated, and the color will be less intense—it will look lighter or fainter. All water color pigments do this, but they do not all to it to the same degree. "Okay," you say, "so you may have to go over a section until you get the intensity you want." Wrong! Part of the inherent beauty of a watercolor painting is the transparency of the medium. Unlike oil or acrylic paintings, light passes through watercolor and reflects from the paper on which the pigment is adhered by gum arabic. By contrast, light reflects off oil and acrylic paint. Going back over a segment of your painting until you get the intensity that you want risks coating the watercolor paper with so much pigment that it becomes opaque at that spot. Thus, at that spot you have caused a different type of light transmission that helps make the eye process that spot differently—a spot that visually is out of place with the rest of the picture. (pp. 249–250)

Just as the meaning of the painting became opaque or impenetrable with repeated strokes of the pen (i.e., the light could no longer penetrate the layers of pigment), the same could be said for families encountering the medical system during the heart murmur discovery and referral. The meaning of the heart murmur as symptom or sign was opaque or ambiguous to the family members. Frawley (1987b), in discussing the semiotics of writing symbols, described this process as he contrasted iconic and opaque representations in various writing systems:

> [Referring to an iconic figure] There is no distinction in the representation between the form of the representation and the meaning represented. In iconic systems, the transparency of the signs allows for no difference between saying and meaning: the saying is the meaning here. In texts, however, there is a distinction between the intention and the form which that intention takes. Opaque signs embody this distinction by definition; the relation between the intention and the expression must be figured out. In less technical terms, transparent representations are self-evident. Texts are not self-evident, but can only become evident. (p. 9)

Recursive Frame Analysis was used to examine interviews with parents so as to illustrate the process by which parents and doctors attempted to make the opaque relationship between the sign of heart murmurs and the meaning of heart murmurs become iconic or transparent. As the framing and the framing of framing unfolded in this interaction, the recursive frame analyst's task, like an epistemologist, "was to mark the orders of recursion invoked in any given description/explanation" (Keeney, 1983, p. 32). "Tracing this recursive operation of drawing distinctions, distinctions upon distinctions and so on, enabled us to uncover the way we constructed and bound together an ecology of ideas—the construction of a reality" (Keeney, 1983, p. 46).

By using the pronouns "us" and "we," Keeney underlined the observing systems nature of Recursive Frame Analysis. Following von Foerster's notion (as cited in Keeney, 1983, pp. 77–78), Keeney pointed out that the act of observing "placed the observer in that which was observed" (p. 77). The same pattern held for this investigation: In the process of carrying out the aesthetical imperative: "If you desire to see, learn how to act" (von Foerster, 1984a, p. 61), this work was constructed.

Therefore, this study was the result of a desire "to see" how parents interpreted the news that one of their children had been diagnosed as having a heart murmur. Learning "how to act" involved an exploration of discourse, narrative, and frame analyses, which helped me to defamiliarize my previous views, so that I could learn "to see" again.

RFA as Method

With the theoretical base now described, the next step is to elaborate on how RFA operates as a research method. One way to help orient readers to the approach RFA investigators take is to examine how RFA relates to another, better-known research method, which shares many of the assumptions inherent in RFA. The other method, the Natural History of an Interview (NHI) (McQuown, 1971c), was arguably the first and most elaborate research method ever applied to the study of human interaction, and it shares many similarities with RFA.

The NHI project was a inter/multidisciplinary investigation which included some of the most brilliant investigators from psychiatry (Frieda Fromm-Reichmann and Henry W. Brosin), linguistics (Charles F. Hockett and Norman A McQuown), anthropology (Gregory Bateson), and kinesics (Ray L. Birdwhistell) (Leeds-Hurwitz, 1987). These researchers were brought together in 1956 by Fromm-Reichmann to produce "a fine-grained analysis, transcription and interpretation of the speech and body motion of participants in a sound-filmed (and tape-recorded) family interview" (McQuown, 1971b, p. 1). Previously, another research group of Fromm-Reichmann had produced a microanalysis of only the speech of participants (McQuown, 1971b, p. 1), but now the group wanted to examine other communication channels (e.g., paralanguage and kinesics) along with speech.

McQuown (1971b) set forth the purpose of the group's investigation of a film provided by Bateson of an interview he had done with a psychiatric patient by stating that NHI was to serve as

> a general introduction to the theory of microanalysis of interviews with a focus on overt behavior, to the individual systems of analysis of the speech and body-motion of participants in such interviews, to the techniques of manipulating taped and filmed materials in order to facilitate such analysis, and to the theoretical frame suitable for the interpretation of the materials and for the use in psychotherapeutic and other practical applications. (p. 2)

Over the next 15-plus years, the original group and other participants produced a five volume work which painstakenly presented: the theoretical background of their study; detailed transcriptions of speech, paralanguage, and kinesics of the Bateson interview; interpretations of the behavior observed in the interview; suggestions for the application of NHI; and numerous appendices which outlined the procedures used to study the interview (McQuown, 1971c). Leeds-Hurwitz (1987) described NHI's importance to the study of communication by stating that NHI

> provided the basis for a view of communication which suggests that it is patterned (non-random, rule-governed, predictable, and therefore analyzable); learned (not inborn, and therefore different for each culture);

> context-bound (behavior has meaning only in a specific context); multichannel (more than just words, communication is a complex combination of words, movements, use of space, etc.); and continuous (it never stops). (p. 31)

NHI directly influenced many other seminal studies of interaction in psychotherapy including *The First Five Minutes: A Sample of Microscopic Interview Analysis* (Pittenger, Hockett, & Danehy, 1960), *Communicational Structure: Analysis of a Psychotherapy Transaction* (Scheflen, 1973), and *Therapeutic Discourse: Psychotherapy as Conversation* (Labov & Fanshel, 1977; Leeds-Hurwitz, 1987). RFA also fits within the research tradition started by the NHI project, but there are some important differences between the two approaches. The similarities and differences between RFA and NHI can best be seen by examining four areas the two methods have in common: (a) How the relationship between context and meaning is presented, (b) how the relationship between micro and macro levels of analysis are understood, (c) how theory is used in the study of overt behavior, and (d) how the study of face-to-face interaction is accomplished. By presenting these comparisons and contrasts, the method of RFA should become readily discernible to the reader.

> RFA was developed to be a precise and concise way of notating the organization of discourse in therapy. Analogous to musical notation, recursive frame analysis enables therapist to immediately visualize the structure, architecture, or anatomy of therapy without engaging in cumbersome theoretical or practical discussions. The method is ideal for both post hoc analyses of whole sessions and as a tool for organizing real-time therapeutic participation in an on-going clinical case. Although recursive frame analysis is principally designed to be a resource for practitioners, it may also contribute to theoretical and research applications. (Keeney, 1990b, pp. 28-29)

From this description, it can be seen that there are two major contexts which have helped to shape RFA. The first influence is that RFA focuses on presenting the organization of discourse in interactions; the second influence is that RFA is designed to be readily accessible to practitioners as well as researchers. Both of these contexts fit well with the NHI approach, but the major contrast between the two approaches centers around the issue of practicality.

NHI stressed practical applications of the method (Leeds-Hurwitz, 1987, p. 18), but the result of the project was a book of dinosaurian proportions. This five volume work was based on analyses of only a few scenes selected from just one film. Similar ratios of talk investigated to length of time involved in the study and size of final presentation of the work (e.g., one session/10 years and over 300 pages of text for Labov and Fanshel's (1977) study), have been the strengths/weaknesses of previous studies. Labov and Fanshel (1977) conceded that a balance had to be found in the study of therapeutic discourse, but that finding harmony between detail and meaning was an arduous task. When speaking of the original NHI project, they wrote

> The wealth of detail and accumulated insights in this unpublished manuscript testifies to the richness of the phenomenon being studied; but it also demonstrates the great difficulty in reducing this information to a parsimonious statement that would allow the knowledge gained to be disseminated broadly and confirmed by other researchers. (p. 20)

Labov and Fanshel made many significant contributions in the evolution of microanalysis of interview processes (e.g., the use of speech acts to analyze therapeutic discourse), but the question of practicality still remained: How can the organization of a session be presented in a meaningful way, without overwhelming the reader and underwhelming the data? Keeney's RFA attempts to address this question. With a focus on creating a system for therapists, which could be used in real-time, RFA was developed to fill a gap between complex methodologies such as NHI, which produce analyses longer than the original works themselves, and unstructured case notes, which may ignore the observable behaviors of the session. NHI was conceived as "a starting point: for further research into analytic and interpretive frames and applications" (Leeds-Hurwitz, 1987, p. 19), and the next sections of this paper will present how RFA can be understood as a logical next phase in well-established tradition.

Context and Meaning

NHI and other microscopic approaches attempt to understand and study interviews in terms of elaborate chainings of successively larger and larger units of analysis which contextualize those levels found below. Bateson (1971) wrote that the NHI team studied "microscopic particles of vocalization towards the most macroscopic units of speech, each step on this ladder is surmounted by placing the units of the lower level in this hierarchy" (p. 16).

How a unit on one level of analysis contextualized or framed units on a lower level was how the NHI investigators studied meaning: " 'Meaning,' therefore, is a function of this restriction of possible meanings" (Bateson, 1971, p. 16).

> This assumption that the microscopic will reflect the macroscopic is a major justification of most of our test procedures. . . . A major function of the techniques of microanalysis is, therefore, to obtain from the small quantities of data, accurately and completely recorded, insights into human relationship which could otherwise only be obtained either by long-term observation or from the notoriously unreliable data of anamnestic reconstruction. (Bateson, 1971, p. 39)

Working from this perspective, these researchers examined how speech, paralanguage, and kinesics were intertwined in human interactions, and how these patterns related to the abstract concepts that were of interest to psychiatry (e.g., transference in the psychoanalytic relationship).

> The ultimate goal of the procedures outlined in this book is a statement of the mechanism of relationships. No statement of mechanism without larger context can be of interest; no statement of relationship, unsubstantiated by a statement of mechanism, can warrant confidence. (Bateson, 1971, p. 40)

The overall purpose and goal of these proceedings was to produce a empirically supportable view of interaction, but the members of the team also realized that reaching such a goal would probably be unattainable.

> Meaning approaches univalence or non-ambiguity only when very large units of the communicational stream are admitted to examination. And even then, the approach to non-ambiguity will be asymptomatic. As larger and larger bodies of data are admitted, the probability of a given interpretation will be increased but proof will never be achieved. The situation is essentially the same as that which obtains in science where no theory is ever proved. (Bateson, 1971, p. 18)

NHI studied units of analysis from the smallest discernable utterances and gestures, to "sentence-like and sentence-sized units" (McQuown, 1971b, p. 4) and recognizable movements such as lighting a cigarette; from strings of sentence-like units and sequences of gestures, to abstract concepts such as "social matrix theories of personality" (McQuown, 1971a, p. 6) and so forth, until the researchers reached an understanding of the meanings of the speech, paralanguage, kinesic, and theoretical structures of the interview.

RFA also focuses on the relationship between smaller units of analysis and larger sequences of behavior, but there are some significant differences in range and width of analysis that occupies the RFA focus. Whereas the NHI investigators were interested in presenting meaning in terms of multichanneled (i.e., speech, kinesic, and paralanguage) contexts, a researcher, working from an RFA perspective, studies how particular utterances are contextualized or understood in terms of previous and subsequent stretches of talk.

For example, consider the following excerpt from a hypothetical therapy session taken from Keeney and Silverstein's (1986) work:

Therapist: Why have you come to therapy?
Client: I hallucinate several times a day.
Therapist: What do you mean, exactly, by "hallucination"?
Client: You know, I hear strange voices that give me secret messages.
Therapist: What do you think these messages mean? (p. 3)

In terms of RFA, the hearing of strange voices is framed or contextualized as being an hallucination, and taken together, these frames contextualize why the client is coming to therapy. These frames would be presented in the following fashion:

Frame (F): Why have you come to therapy?
  Frame (F): I hallucinate several times a day.
    Frame (F): I hear strange voices that give me secret messages.

The indentation is meant to represent how certain frames are understood as being framed by other frames. But it is important to remember that, although the "strange voices" frame is represented as being embedded within the "hallucination" frame, this is not to infer that there is a dependent/independent relationship between the two frames. Following Bateson's (1972) comments as elaborated above, the "strange voices" are understood in terms of being referred to as "hallucinations," as well as being part of the hallucinations.

The therapeutic importance of being able to make that distinction is that it provides the clinician with a number of ways to approach therapy with this client. One approach would entail exploring the client's willingness to accept another framing for the strange voices, other than that of hallucinations. Another avenue to explore would be to examine what other behavior is also framed by the client as being either hallucinations, or worthy of therapeutic intervention. Still another possibility is to investigate times and situations during which hearing strange voices which give the client secret messages is a resource for the client.

All of these potential moves by the clinician are intended to create shifts in the client's talk. These changes in talk may lead to changes in behavior for the client such that previous problematic situations no longer exist for the client, or if the situations do continue, they are no longer framed as being worrisome or in need of therapeutic intrusion.

For a researcher investigating therapeutic discourse, RFA can be used to chart the shifts or lack of shifts in the talk. For example, if the therapist from the above mentioned example offered a new frame for the client's hearing of strange voices, the researcher would be interested in charting how the introduction of the new frame was used by the client. In addition, the researcher could investigate if the client's use of the therapist's framing helped to shift the talk out of the context of hearing strange voices is a reason to be in therapy.

Therapist: Have you ever considered that the voices you hear are real and not imagined hallucinations?

Client: Yes. My mother used to hear voices too and she said that they were from angels.

If the client acknowledges that the voices are real hallucinations (i.e., They are messages from angelic sources.), then that represents a possible shift in the therapeutic conversation. Rather than talking about medicating the client for hearing imagined voices, the therapist can begin to explore how hearing angels' voices like mother did, makes sense within the context of the client. For example, it may be discovered, that the client believes that hearing voices like mother is a way for the client to remain loyal to that parent. If this is so, then the therapist may help the client come up with a new way to be loyal to mother without having to hear voices. A researcher could follow the therapist-client discourse throughout the course of therapy to see how the talk was framed and reframed, or how meaning was constructed, reconstructed, and deconstructed.

Whereas NHI studied meaning in terms of phonemes, sentences, and other linguistic, parlinguistic, and kinesic units of analysis, RFA focuses on meaning in the talk in terms of how certain utterances can be understood to frame or be framed by other utterances. The differences between how microscopic the analyses NHI and RFA is determined by the question, "How low must one go in the course of microanalysis in order to feel confident that the assumptions made at a higher level are properly substantiated by the units of a lower level?"

For RFA, the answer is that words can be understood in terms of other words. In order to present discourse in a manageable, yet meaningful fashion, the RFA therapist or researcher uses distinctions drawn in the talk of the participants, to describe that same talk. The process of RFA is akin to that of musical notation: Musical notes are understood or heard in terms of other musical notes. A note played in one chord, produces a sound different than the same note played in a different chord. Keeney (Keeney & Ross, 1985) described this note/chord relationship by sharing an anecdote about the jazz pianist, Oscar Peterson:

> Oscar Peterson . . . was once asked how he feels when he hits an occasional wrong note. He replied that "since every note can be related to a chord," there can be no wrong notes. The trick is to integrate whatever note you happen to hit into one's musical arrangement. (pp. 126–127)

For the RFA researcher, the trick is to demonstrate how each note (or frame) was integrated into the musical arrangement (or discourse) that is being studied. The goal of this process is to score the conversation such that another reader (or listener) could come along at a later time, and not only follow, but also appreciate the note progressions and various chord changes that constituted the piece studied.

Another similarity between NHI and RFA is on the role theory plays in the investigation of discourse. To this concern, Bateson (1971) wrote

> We start from a particular interview on a particular day between two identified persons in the presence of a child, a camera and a cameraman. Our primary data are the multitudinous details of vocal and bodily action recorded on this film. We call our treatment of such data a "natural history" because a minimum of theory guided the collection of data. (p. 6)

The same could be said for RFA: As a method of investigation, RFA is based upon cybernetic notions of recursion, feedback, and calibration (see Keeney, 1983). These assumptions help to guide the therapist or the researcher in searching and researching the talk at hand. When used in the course of conducting systemic family therapy, the charting of frames can be done independent of any particular orientation to therapy. The idea that an utterance can be understood with a context of another set of words is not dependent on a school of therapy, but rather on the notion that communication can be understood in terms of context and embeddedness.

When applied to research, the same relationship between the observations made, and the theory used to make those distinctions: The charting of frames can be done independent of any social or psychological theory of face-to-face interaction. Of course, another researcher may read an RFA of an interaction and cite the configuration of frames as a demonstration of a particular theory of interaction (e.g., dramatic scripting) (Goffman, 1974). But, that particular punctuation of behavior reflects a relationship between the observer's conceptualization and the frames presented, and not necessarily anything within the RFA analysis itself.

Procedures and Process

The final comparison to be made between NHI and RFA is the process by which each investigation is carried out. Although the two methods may differ as to the levels and channels of analysis studied, the process of the investigations is similar. Investigations from a NHI perspective involve a three step sequence: soaking (i.e., multiple viewing-listening of the film and/or tape of the interview), scene selection (i.e., after numerous viewings, select sequences of behavior), and intensive analysis (i.e., transcribe and closely examine the overt behavior) (Leeds-Hurwitz, 1987, p. 8).

The process of RFA differs slightly depending on the purpose for which it is being used. For use during a particular therapeutic sessions, there is not time for elaborate soakings and intensive analysis, but if RFA is used to study interviews such as the ones recorded for this study, the process resembles that of NHI. The RFA investigator repeatedly listens/watches the video/audiotape in order to transcribe the session. Following Hopper's (1988, p. 54) suggestion, the reading of the transcript is always associated with the playing of the actual tape of the session. The purpose is that reading the transcript along with listening to the tape allows the researcher ample opportunities to improve the transcription. If the tape is ignored, the transcript of the session can never be improved.

As the transcription is being made and remade, the RFA researcher begins to chart the frames of the interview. Certain sequences of the talk (e.g., words, phrases, etc.) are notated as frames. As was the case with the therapy example given above, words such as *hallucinations* and *strange voices* were distinguished as frames to be considered for further study. The choice of these frames is done in a discovery-oriented fashion.

The next step in the sequence is to begin to group frames so as to represent how frames are being contextualized by other frames. As was done with the previous therapy excerpt, the frame of strange voices was indicated to be understood in terms of an hallucination, and that both of those frames were represented as being understood by the observer as being contextualized by the therapy frame. Different orders of frames (i.e., frames that include other frames) can be called *galleries* (Keeney, in press). For example, the talk in the previous excerpt could be said to have occurred within a gallery of therapy.

Shifts in the discourse are marked. These shifts, called openings (Keeney, in press), are notations that represent that the talk has moved from one context to another. Again, returning to the therapy example given above, the therapist and client interaction centering around the voices being from angels may be an opening out of the frame of hallucinations and into the frame of alternative explanations for the voices. The researcher would have to track the sequence of frames in order to observe that the talk had indeed moved from the context of hallucination. As was the case with Oscar Peterson's "wrong note," the meaning of a frame can not be understood in isolation apart from the other utterances. Each frame is understood as being a part of the rest of the discourse.

This process of transcript improvement, frame identification, and frame relating continues throughout the investigation of the talk. In the case of the study of the talk for this research, the structure of the interviews provided certain pre-discourse galleries to be investigated. For example, the interviewers had certain prearranged galleries or topics that were to be asked to the parents (e.g., How was the heart murmur discovered?). When that gallery was introduced by the interviewer, the researcher could then chart the frames that were elicited by the heart murmur discovery question. Was the discovery framed by the parents as being routine, or was the identification of the child's murmur contextualized as being problematic or worthy of worry?

Galleries such as the discovery of the heart murmur, the parents' expectations of seeing the pediatric cardiologist, and changes in how the child was being treated now that the heart murmur had been discovered could be compared from parent interview to parent interview. This would allow the investigator to see how the talk in those galleries was similar and/or different for each parent interviewed. For example, when parents were asked about their expectations of seeing the heart specialist, the researcher would be interested in noting how parents contextualized the consultation: Was the meeting framed as being the final, positive answer for the parents, or was the face-to-face encounter being treated as another in a long line of potential disappointments?

It would be important to know how parents may possibly contextualize different aspects of the heart murmur discovery-referral process. Given the relationship between utterances and the context in which they may be understood, physicians and parents both may benefit from an investigation such as this one. A physician's talk about a child's heart can be understood in many ways. Having a way to study the process by which meanings are negotiated during interactions would be invaluable to understanding doctor-patient communication and miscommunication. RFA is meant to be another contribution to the process started by NHI: "Such application will inevitably lead to the refinement both of the descriptive tools and of the interpretive frames with which descriptive results are evaluated" (McQuown, 1971a, p. 10). In the next chapter, this process of RFA investigation is discussed further in terms of the methods and procedures employed in the study of the parents' talk about their children's heart murmurs.

Chapter 3
Method

INTRODUCTION

This chapter presents the details of the research process employed in this project. Special emphasis was placed on elaborating the means by which the organization of the parents' talk was analyzed, and how these procedures helped to shape the investigation and reporting of the parents' accounts of their experiences surrounding the discovery of their child's heart murmur, and the subsequent referral of the child to a pediatric cardiologist.

SUBJECTS AND PROCEDURES

This study was based upon analysis of 32 interviews with families of children referred by a primary care physician to the cardiology unit of a major medical complex. Each interview was conducted during the family's first visit, just prior to the family's consultation with the cardiology specialist. After the family had checked into the clinic and the child had been taken to the radiology unit for x-rays, had been given an EKG, and had been examined by a nurse from the cardiology unit, the family was introduced to an interviewer. Four doctoral students from the marriage and family therapy program at Texas Tech University, who were identified as "counselors," conducted these interviews. The interviews were done over a two and one-half month period. Families were selected based upon the following: (a) this appointment being their first appointment at the cardiology unit, and (b) the availability of the interviewer. The interviewers would check with the intake receptionist at least two times per week to determine when new patients were scheduled. Nevertheless, some patients were seen in the clinic when no interviewer was available.

The timing of these interviews was significant in that the cardiologist's diagnosis had not yet been made at the time of these interviews. Since the diagnosis was unknown but was imminent, the families' worries could be expected to be most intense at that point in the process.

To commence the process, interviewers presented an overview of the research for the family, then requested and obtained their written permission to participate in this study. Permission was then obtained to audiotape these interviews. Next, the interviewers administered a brief questionnaire, and then conducted the interview. Each of these interviews lasted approximately 20 minutes.

The intent of the interviews was to determine (a) the family members' understanding of their experience with the primary care physician in regard to how the heart murmur was discussed and how the decision for referral was made, (b) the family members' concerns about the heart murmur diagnosis, and (c) the family members' expectations of their consultation with the pediatric cardiologist.

ANALYSIS

The analysis of these interviews involved a style of discourse analysis similar to the method suggested by Potter and Wetherell (1987). Key to this method are procedures for transcription and analysis. These transcripts are somewhat more detailed than typical ones employed in discourse analysis, though not as detailed as the transcripts of recent conversation analysis (Freeman, 1987). The following guidelines for transcription were observed: Transcribe all words as they were spoken, indicate noticeable pauses by placing a period in parentheses, mark overlapped utterances using brackets to indicate portions that overlap, and indicate salient paralinguistic features as laughter (in parentheses) and intonation (by use of periods to show falling intonation and question marks for rising intonation). Unintelligible portions of the tape were represented by double parentheses). After transcription, the typed transcript and audiotape were compared to monitor and improve accuracy (see Hopper, 1988).

The analysis of the interviews was not aimed at understanding the organization of discourse solely in terms of the interactional structure between the interviewers and the interviewees. The interaction was understood as being a narrative, and by focusing on the conversation as narrative, the investigator was allowed to consider the different aspects of a narrative's structure: event and evaluative structures, and explanatory systems (Linde, 1986, pp. 186–190). An event structure consisted of the "the 'facts' of the narrative" (Linde, 1986, p. 186). The evaluative structure involved "the means by which the speaker conveyed to the addressees how the event structure was to be understood: loosely speaking, what the events meant to the speaker" (Linde, 1986, pp. 186–187). The explanatory system was taken to mean "the system of assumptions about the world which the speaker used to make events and evaluations coherent'' (Linde, 1986, p. 188). These explanatory systems could be derived from ''common sense,'' or from so-called ''expert systems'' such as psychological explanatory systems (e.g., ''Freudian'' or ''behavioral'') (Linde, 1986, p. 189–190).

Investigation of narrative structure provided a way to discern variability in how families characterized the event in which referral took place, how they described their concerns for their children, and what expectations they voiced for resolution of their crisis by pediatric cardiologists. Accordingly, the first determination was in regards to what each family had said about the context of referral, their concerns, and their expectations. As is typical of this sort of analysis, many of families' utterances bridged two of these categories, as when a family member explained that she became worried when the referring physician made the appointment with the specialist himself, rather than relying on the parents to do so.

As the work progressed, there was increased interest in the ''small details'' of how referrals were made, and what these nuances meant to families in terms of how they understood the event of referral, how concerned they became, and how their expectations were generated. For instance, in the example alluded to in the previous paragraph, the referring doctor himself led the family to understand the event as a serious and urgent medical problem, as opposed to a benign anomaly the child would have probably grown out of naturally.

When analyzing talk, an investigator has many choices as far as how the structure of the discourse is to be studied and presented. Schwartz and Jacobs (1979, p. 342) discussed five possible approaches to the examination of the layers of organization in conversations or narratives: the turn-taking system (i.e., how speakers take and relinquish the floor during conversations); the recursive organization (i.e., how previous utterances determine how to listen to and how to produce a current utterance); overall structural organization (i.e., how conversations begin and end); intra-utterance structure (i.e., what singular utterances accomplish in the talk); and interconversational structure (i.e., how speakers relate entire conversations to other conversations).

In this investigation, special attention was paid to two types of organizations in the parents' talk: intra-utterance structure and recursive organization. The intra-utterance analysis focused on pragmatics by examining the use of such speech acts as aligning actions (Stokes & Hewitt, 1976), accounts (Scott & Lyman, 1968), and disclaimers (Hewitt & Stokes, 1975). Speech acts can be best understood as the study of how people do things with words; that is, how do people accomplish desired actions, such as making excuses, through the use of words in conversation (Urmson & Sbisa, 1975; Potter & Wetherell, 1987). For example, in the talk studied for this project, special attention was paid to how parents gave accounts so as to create contexts in which it made sense for an expert like a doctor to not know what was wrong with their child.

The examination of recursive organization of the parents' narratives was conducted from a Recursive Frame Analysis (RFA) perspective (Keeney, 1987b, 1990a, 1990b). The process of RFA entailed the following procedures: (a) note frames elicited during the interviews with the families; (b) sort frames in a discovery-oriented manner (e.g., Mahrer, 1988) in terms of frame sequence (i.e., trace the succession of frames in the narratives) and frame embeddedness (i.e., sketch how frames contextualize each other in the discourse); (c) mark groupings of frames, otherwise known as gallery boundaries, and name them (i.e., show how frames were connected, or how talk in a sequence was more of the same); (d) look for openings (i.e., highlight differences in the talk, which may or may not have keyed shifts in the conversations); (e) indicate doors (i.e., mark frames which represented shifts in talk from one gallery to another); and (f) look for markers or rims of frames (Goffman, 1974) (i.e., note information supplied by the speakers which gave indication as to how a frame should be understood).

The procedures were continued for each of the family interviews. RFAs, created from the interviews, were then related to each other so as to compare and contrast different families' frames and galleries on similar topics. For example, in the area of heart murmur discovery, how similar or different were the families' accounts of their experiences surrounding the heart murmur identification which lead to the referral to the pediatric cardiologist?

The investigation of intra-utterance and recursive organizations was structured in the following manner: (a) focus on exemplars, which constitute and support the distinctions being made; (b) compare and contrast prior exemplars with subsequent examplars; (c) explore similarities/differences between these exemplars; and (d) present the exemplars such that initial examples serve as prototypes, and subsequent illustrations demonstrate variability within a specific distinction (Potter & Wetherell, 1987, pp. 122-123). In addition to these considerations, an investigator would display the exemplar with "as much of its surrounding talk as possible—preferably the entire conversation" (Schwartz & Jacobs, 1979, p. 343).

Although the range of material covered in this study prohibits presenting complete parent interviews, every attempt would be made so that each exemplar chosen would be accompanied by as much of the surrounding talk as possible. These efforts to contextualize the exemplars would be consistent with how conversation or discourse analysts "take pains to re-present data richly. Conversation-analytic data reductions occur late in inquiry, and their results appear in choices of exemplars, and specifications of their details in prose description" (Hopper, 1988, p. 57). But at the same time, there is the need to preserve enough of the conversation, from which the exemplar was pulled, so that the examples' discourse ecology is well represented.

The aesthetics of discourse analysis involves the relationship between the parts chosen from the conversation, and that conversation in its entirety. With that relationship, the discourse analyst must also balance the dilemma of presenting an ideal quantity of exemplars so that the reader can grasp the rule or concept being discussed, without being overwhelmed or bored by the sheer number of examples. With each investigation, the struggle begins anew. "The conversation analysts' art includes examining a number of instances in the context of discovery, but reporting only a few of these in scientific essays, accompanying each reported case with detailed description" (Hopper, 1988, p. 57). What constitutes "a few" is always debatable.

As for testing the reliability and validity of the claims made in the presentation of examples, the sequence followed in this project adhered to a falsification process as described by Hopper (1988) and McQuown (1971a). Although these ways to access testability differ from the methods employed in experimental studies, it does not mean that the discourse analysts ignore questions of accountability in their investigations (see Potter & Wetherell, 1987, pp. 66–71, 159).

Hopper (1988) has described a process by which the conversation or discourse analyst tests and retests the ways in which the organization of talk is being construed.

> Conversation analysts approach falsification by testing descriptions against the details of each new instance. Sometimes a counter-instance invalidates or transforms an analysis. . . . Sometimes a counter-instance stimulates a modification of a rule or may be described in terms of interactions of phenomena. Sometimes a counter-instance aids an analyst by showing how participants react to violation. There are few transcendent rules for falsification in conversation analysis. (Hopper, 1988, p. 56)

As each new transcript and tape was examined, new distinctions were compared to previous ones. In a sense, what Hopper was writing about was the notion of reliability: Through repeated measures or examinations, how reliable are the observations or distinctions which have been drawn by the observer? The task of the analyst is to continually reexamine and research the text or talk being studied. The purpose of this recycling is for the investigator to rigorously test the findings of the study by constantly comparing the results to the data.

Once the investigator chooses the examples and accompanies them with concise descriptions, these findings are presented for other investigators to peruse. The purpose of these presentations is to allow others to validate the observations made by the initial investigator. McQuown (1971a) outlined this validation process in his summary of *The Natural History of an Interview:*

> Uncertain though our interpretations of behavior might be, we may now produce a corpus of specified behavioral phenomena on which such interpretations are based, a corpus which is available to all for repeated examination for correction where correction is demonstrably necessary, for refinement where refinement is desired, and for the testing of new interpretive hypotheses where the old ones have proven to be unjustifiable. (p. 8)

The purpose, then, is: (a) to present distinctions drawn from the talk of parents about their child's heart murmur, (b) to accompany these distinctions with surrounding talk from the interviews so as to provide needed context, (c) to supply descriptions or rationales for these distinctions, and (d) to allow readers the opportunity to judge the validity of the conclusions drawn from the talk. This mode of presentation allows for the type of refinement that McQuown (1971a) suggested above.

In Chapter 4, what was taken to be the most pronounced features of families' understandings of the context of referral and their concerns about their children will be displayed. Part of what made these features prominent was the poignancy of their expressions, something that would not have been revealed in other sorts of research into this problem. Also, however, this analysis indicated a number of points of divergence between the medical view of referral that was reviewed above, and the experiences of the families interviewed. These, too, were salient features to be displayed.

Chapter 4
Analysis and Interpretation

INTRODUCTION

The analysis in this chapter is presented through three, intertwining threads: (a) exemplars (Hopper, 1988) chosen to represent distinctions discovered in or constructed from the 32 family interviews, (b) descriptive passages which attempt to highlight the distinctions found in the exemplars and illustrate relationships between different exemplars and between exemplars and points made in the literature, and (c) Recursive Frame Analysis (RFA) (Keeney, 1990a, 1990b) passages which attempt to describe the distinctions drawn in the interaction between the interview exemplars and the descriptive paragraphs. None of the threads have hierarchy over the other two: Each informs the others and are, in turn, informed by the others. The three strands are woven together to produce a pattern which strives to represent the stories of the families in the study. The tales are the families' interpretations of their experiences during the referral process to a pediatric cardiologist. For all of the families, the reason for referral to a heart specialist is the same: A child in the family has been diagnosed as having a heart murmur. The following is a presentation of these stories.

The subsequent exemplars were chosen from various transcripts of the family interviews. Certain conventions were used in the presentation of these exemplars: (a) Names of the speakers and medical personnel were deidentified so as to protect their confidentiality, (b) abbreviations were used to designate the speakers (M for the mother, F for the father, and I for the interviewer), (c) material inserted into the exemplars to show emphasis (i.e., italics added), or to expand the utterances so as to make the meanings clearer (i.e., in the cases of indexicality or ellipsis) were placed in brackets.

DISCOVERY AND REFERRAL

The first part of each interview focused on how family members discovered or became aware of their child's possible heart murmur. In analyzing the interviews, two distinct patterns of discovery emerged.

For some families, the heart murmur was first identified during the medical consult which lead to the referral to the pediatric cardiologist. These discoveries took place under varying circumstances: during football physicals, regularly scheduled checkups, and appointments for other illnesses such as ear infections.

Excerpt A

(01) *I:* Okay a a few questions just to kind of begin is what happened
(02) that brought you here today with your son?
(03) *F:* Well he went to take a physical to play football [the doctor
(04) discovered he had] a little heart murmur.

Excerpt B

(01) *I:* So when you took uh Susie to Dr. Girardi, he was doing I guess a
(02) three-week check up maybe.
(03) *M:* Yeah, two weeks.
(04) *I:* . . . So what did he tell you?
(05) *M:* Her heart was beating too fast.

While the discovery in the last example (B) came early in the child's life (at "a three-week check up"), for some families (Excerpt C), the heart murmur was discovered even sooner while their child was a newborn and was still in the hospital after delivery.

Excerpt C

(01) *M:* Well, uh, when he was born the pediatrician was on call (.)
(02) noticed a small heart murmur and said it was a small hole in the
(03) back of (( )) chamber and he just wanted us to check it out and
(04) made an appointment and that's what we are here (.) just
checking it out.

For other families, there had been prior knowledge of irregularities in their child's heart, but the identification of a heart murmur represented a change from a previous diagnosis. Excerpt D was from a mother who had noticed that her son had "an irregular heartbeat." She had made her discovery while playing with a stethoscope the family owned. Her son had had a couple of appointments over several months and none of the medical personnel had mentioned anything about her son's irregular heartbeat. In the quote, the mother tells how "irregular heartbeat" was rediagnosed as "heart murmur."

Excerpt D

(01) *M:* . . . and so this time I asked the doctor myself, I said it has never
(02) been brought to my attention I said but he does have an irregular
(03) beat. And she says "well it's just a murmur" and I said "well I've
(04) never been (.) told that he had a heart murmur"

In contrast to these families, other families had knowledge of a heart murmur prior to the medical consult with the referring physician.

Excerpt E

(01) *I:* What's your understanding of what is going on with Tim?
(02) *M:* I really don't know, his doctor just told me, his pediatrician, that
(03) . . . visible at school. . . Tim has bad knees and all . . . said that
(04) she heard a click, and she said that it may be due to his chest
(05) kind of goes in, and she said that sometimes this happens, she
(06) didn't think it was anything serious but she wanted it checked
(07) he's had a heart murmur when he was smaller, he was born with
(08) one but that accounts for . . . she called it a micro . . . valve or
(09) something like that, I don't know.

Excerpt E illustrated some aspects of the discovery process that were common to many of the families interviewed: The families questioned their knowledge of what was happening with their child: "*I really don't know*, [italics added] his doctor just told me" and "she called it a micro . . . valve or *something like that, I don't know*" [italics added] and they seemed to be caught up in a "yes, but" -type of experience: "she didn't think it was anything serious *but* [italics added] she wanted it checked out."

Excerpt F was another example of the "yes, but" scenario: "she [the doctor] didn't say it was anything serious *but* [italics added] she thought that maybe it's just a good idea to go ahead and check it out . . ." The last part of the mother's statement was also interesting. Although some families had considerable exposure to heart-related medical care, others had neither the personal/familial nor the medical context from which to understand the current happenings. For this mother, there appeared to be little prior contact ("I I never had anything like that happen to my kids") that would have helped her during the discovery/referral procedures.

Excerpt F

(01) *I:* What did Doctor Carter say at the time (( )) she presented to you
(02) (.)
(03) *M:* Well she didn't say that it was anything serious but she thought
(04) that maybe she it's just a good idea to go ahead and check it out
(05) (( )) see what's going wrong it's gonna be I I never had anything
(06) like that happen to my kids

In Excerpt G, the mother described how she had her husband call the doctor the evening the referral decision was made. The mother and/or father were not sure that the mother had correctly understood the doctor's rationale for referral: "I wanted to know for sure I had not misinterpreted anything she [the doctor] had told [me]. . ."

Excerpt G

(01) *I:* Okay, so what your husband knows is what you reported to him?
(02) *M:* Yeah. Well he also talked with the doctor. He called her that
(03) evening and they discussed Tim also.
(04) *I:* Okay . . . you wanted to find out more or what . . .
(05) *M:* Well, I wanted to know for sure I had not misinterpreted anything
(06) she had told . . . you know . . .

Like the mother in Excerpt G, many parents discussed their sense of not knowing whether they understood either the diagnosis and/or the decision whether or not to refer. In Excerpt H, the mother demonstrated her lack of certainty concerning the diagnosis: "he [the doctor] called it a benign murmur *that is what I'm thinking* [italics added]" and "That the blood *might* [italics added] be rushing too fast. . ." This hesitancy or hedging was understandable given that she had not heard the conclusive word from the cardiologist. But what was also curious in the quote, was how she recalled the doctor's use of a *disclaimer* (Hewitt & Stokes, 1975): "but he [the doctor] said I don't know." Hewitt and Stokes (1975) described as "an interactional tactic employed by actors faced with upcoming events or acts which threatened to disrupt emergent meanings and discredit cathected identities" (p. 1). By qualifying his statement with an utterance such as he used, the doctor could have been preserving his identity as a doctor (i.e., an expert): He was such an expert that he could predict when he was going to be wrong. If his diagnosis turned out to be correct, then the disclaimer could have been dismissed as being a necessary caution.

Excerpt H

(01) *I:* Did they talk to you about it?
(02) *P:* Briefly (.) I asked them what it was and they told me that the
(03) sound makes my heart go boom boom uh okay
(04) *I:* So they explained
(05) *M:* he called it a benign murmur that is what I'm thinking
(06) *I:* Oh
(07) *M:* That the blood might be rushing through too fast but he said I
(08) don't know

With some of the discovery sequences, such as the one illustrated in Excerpt H, there seemed to be an interaction of dual unbalancing acts. On one hand, the family members were introduced to new information which altered the ways in which they viewed their child: a child with no heart murmur to a child with a heart murmur. The discovery of a heart murmur unsettled or unbalanced the status quo for many families interviewed in the study. On the other hand, the referring physicians were not so certain of the heart murmur's innocent nature. If the doctors were certain of the insignificance of the murmur, they would not have referred the family to the heart specialist. The referring physicians, like the families, were also in a knowing/not knowing oscillation.

Another possible, complicating factor in the discovery to referral workings was the rapidity of the process. The quick pace at which the proceedings were sometimes carried out could be seen in Excerpt I. With this family, the physician who originally discovered the heart murmur was also the doctor who subsequently referred the family to a specialist.

Excerpt I

(01) *I:* The sixteenth. Okay. And then how soon after did Dr. Carlisle
(02) discover the murmur.
(03) *M:* Okay. That same day she came in and told us that she thought
(04) there was one. And then had us an appointment for the next day
(05) at her office to come in there. And she heard it again and let us
(06) listen to it.

After running a few more tests, the doctor then referred the family to the pediatric cardiologist. The discovery/referral time frame for this family was quite rapid. The child was born on a Tuesday. The murmur was first discovered that same day. The child was reexamined on Wednesday. Tests were run on Friday and the child was seen by the cardiologist that Monday; six days from birth to visiting a heart specialist.

Excerpt J also showed the swift turnaround faced by some families:

Excerpt J

(01) *M:* He didn't. He just said, "When can you go to Lubbock?" I said,
(02) "Tomorrow if I have to." (laughter)
(03) *I:* When was this?
(04) *M:* Thursday.
(05) *F:* Thursday.
(06) *I:* Okay so it was as soon as you could come that you did come.
(07) *M:* Um hum.

As stated above, the rapid pace of the referral workings, as experienced by some families, was indeed bewildering. In addition to the rate at which the families had to assimilate the considerable flow of information, there was also the question of the symbolic meaning the prompt calling for referral had for the families. At one instance, the doctor was describing the murmur as being inconsequential, while at the same time, the referral sequence was being carried out at a rapid rate. Of course, for some families, the process was not being completed quickly enough:

Excerpt K

(01) *M:* Really our family life hasn't changed, you know . . uh . . I try the
(02) worrying I do . . I try to do by myself . . and uh . . as far as the
(03) worse thing I can think of . . this is probably so minor is the way
(04) . . you know . . this right here [coming to the heart specialist], its
(05) really getting to me (laughter) . . you know cause I'm here and I
(06) want to find out what's wrong and I want it yesterday . . that's
(07) my problem.

Another contrast between the families during the discovery process was the amount of investigating that was completed by the referring physician prior to the referral being made. For some of the families in the study, the physician detected the murmur with the use of a stethoscope and then made the decision to refer the child. Tests, commonly used in the confirmation of an innocent heart murmur such as a chest X ray or electrocardiogram (ECG) (Kiester, Jr., 1982), were not conducted.

Excerpt L

(01) *F:* Well, he recommended us to come out here. If he ran a test up
(02) there, he had to send us here anyway.

But for other families, standard tests such as the ECG were carried out and the family was still referred to the cardiologist.

Excerpt M

(01) *F:* we took her to the doctor cause of that ear infection right
(02) *M:* Mm hmm
(03) *F:* and then there they did some tests on em and they said she had a
(04) heart murmur

Excerpt N

(01) *M:* . . . they ran they ran an EKG and some x-rays there. She said
(02) that she thought it [the murmur] looked fine but she'd rather a
(03) cardiologist look at it.

For families like the two of these, the referring physician went beyond the stethoscope in order to diagnose the heart murmur. But in both cases, the doctors were still unable to make a definitive statement without the input from a heart specialist: "She [the doctor] said she thought it [the murmur] looked fine *but* [italics added] she'd rather a cardiologist look at it."

As was seen in these discovery scenarios, the process varied from family to family in terms of prior knowledge of the heart murmur, period of time between discovery and referral, and reason for seeing the eventual referring physician. Despite these differences in discovery, the families in this study had one common characteristic: They all had a child with a heart murmur that was worthy of referral to a pediatric cardiologist.

RFA of Discovery and Referral

As was discussed in the previous chapter, RFA was used to describe the parents' talk about their experiences with referring physicians and other concerned parties because RFA was a way to present interaction-in-context (Keeney, in press). The recursive relationship between interaction and context was brought into focus by the simple action of drawing distinctions (Spencer-Brown, 1972). The observer or, in this case, the researcher drew distinctions (frames) to understand how the parents organized their interactions-in-context.

To illustrate the distinctions drawn in the parents' talk, the following RFA conventions were used:

1. Upper- and lower-case letters *F/f* were used to designate a word or group of words as a *frame* (e.g., F: She didn't think it was anything serious.). The lower case f was used to demonstrate that one frame (f) was taken to be embedded within another frame (F):

F: She didn't think it was anything serious.
    f: she heard a click.

The configuring of the preceding frames would represent that the hearing of the click was meant to be understood as not being anything serious.

2. An upper-case letter G was used to represent a word or group of words as a *gallery* (e.g., G: Healthy child). Numbers were used with the upper case G's to represent shifts in the discourse from one context or gallery to another context or gallery:

G1: Healthy child
G2: Unhealthy child.

Frames listed under a gallery were meant to designate that those frames were to be understood within the context of that gallery:

G1: Routine Check up
    F: Routine referral.

The configuration of the preceding gallery and frame represented that the frame of routine referral was meant to be understood within the context of the routine check up gallery.

3. Indentation was meant to represent embeddedness of frames and galleries:

G1: Routine Check up
  F: Listening to heart
    f: Hearing heart murmur.

The preceding configuration represented that the hearing heart murmur frame was meant to be understood within the context or frame of listening to the heart, and both of these frames were meant to be understood within the larger, encompassing context or gallery of routine checkups.

By using the conventions outlined above, the RFA researcher was interested in portraying ways in which families framed the discovery of the heart murmur and how they contextualized the ongoing interaction with the doctors. The process folded back upon itself as the discovery of the parent of new or different information about their child's heart lead to their (re)contextualization of the ongoing medical process.

Each new discovery made by the parents lead to new (re)contextualizations of the ongoing medical process. A focus on a circular organization of contextualizing-interacting-(re)contextualizing helped the researcher to begin to understand a context in which the concerns by parents made sense and, in other instances, contexts in which the lack of concerns by parents also made sense.

For some families in the study, the process of discovery/referral began during a routine medical check up (Gallery 1, or simply G1). From a context or gallery of a usual doctor's appointment, the parents had had certain expectations or frames (F) which they anticipated during the examination:

G1: Routine Medical Checkup
  F1: Listen to heart   F2: Listen to lungs
  F3: Look at eyes   F4: Look at ears

With the families who had no prior knowledge of any irregularities, the gallery of routine checkup included an unexpected frame (f): a heart murmur.

G1: Routine Medical Checkup
  F1: Listen to heart
    f: "a little heart murmur" (Excerpt A)
    f: "Her heart was beating too fast" (Excerpt B)

f: "noticed a small heart murmur" (Excerpt C)
f: "a small hole in the back ((   )) chamber" (Excerpt C)

Given the discovery of these new frames (f's), the families could have questioned the initial gallery of *routine* medical encounter.

G1a: Routine Medical Checkup
    F1: Listen to heart
        f: Hear heart murmur.
            G1b: Routine Medical Checkup ?

As new information was added, the resiliency of the context (Tannen & Wallat, 1986) as being routine was tested. Maisede (1987, p. 68) called this process "permanent context construction" or "the indexicality of context." By this, Maisede meant "that while the ongoing interaction depends on social context, it simultaneously generates, reproduces, and changes the context" (p. 68). The permanent context construction of Maisede contrasted well with what Keeney (1983) described as the nature of circularity, repetition or pattern:

> These terms suggest that ideas, experience, and social events do more than stretch out in lineal time. When a process folds upon itself, we speak of recursion. The image of a circle is probably not the best way to think of recursion since we are not really referring to an original beginning point in time. *Each recursive loop does imply a different beginning, although in terms of the pattern of organization, it is simply recycled* [italics added]. (pp. 58–59)

Following this line of reasoning, each time the family received new information about their child's heart, the gallery of routine was/could have been questioned. If the context of routine medical procedures was/could have been maintained by the doctors and the families, then succeeding frames such as more tests, more exams, and referral were/would have been understood as being routine. If the context of routine medical procedures was not/could not have been maintained, then the subsequent moves of more tests and referral were/would have been contextualized as being something other than routine.

For each family in the study, the question became, "Did the gallery of routine medical encounter fit with the frames being presented during the visit with the doctor?" Agar (1985, p. 149) described this process as the interaction between institutional frames and client frames. In the discourse collected in this study, there were examples of parents' and doctors' attempts to maintain the gallery of routine.

There were numerous instances where parents and physicians helped each other maintain the routineness of the process. In Excerpt

D, Line 03, the mother recalled the doctor's phrasing of the murmur discovery: "And she says 'well it's *just* a murmur' " [italics added]. The use of the word "just" when she announced the discovery of the murmur, could have been a way for the doctor to help maintain a gallery of routineness by framing the condition in a *matter-of-fact* fashion.

Other ways in which the doctors framed the discovery and referral as being routine/non-problematic were evident in Excerpts C and E. In RFA terms, Excerpt C was understood as follows:

G1: "The pediatrician was on call." (routine)
  F: "noticed a small heart murmur"
    f: "he wanted us to check it out and made an appointment"
      G2: "we are here (.) just checking it out" (routine)

G2 was represented as being embedded in G1 because the mother seemed to maintain the theme (Agar, 1979) of routine. The pediatrician on call (routine) wanted the parents to have the *small* heart murmur checked out (routine) and the parents did just that ("we are here (.) just checking it out") (routine).

In Excerpt E, the doctor's attempt to frame the discovery as being routine or nonproblematic had a leak (Keeney, 1990a) in it. At first the doctor framed the discovery of the heart murmur as being nonserious.

F: She didn't think it was anything serious.
  f: she heard a click.

Then the mother recalled the doctor saying, "but she wanted it checked out." That phrase could have been taken as another frame contextualized by the previous frame, i.e., the heart murmur was not anything serious, or the use of the word "but" could have helped to create a side-by-side construction.

F: She didn't think it was anything serious
/BUT/
F: She wanted it checked out.

The use of the word "but" helped to create two possible contexts: one characterized as being nonserious; the other characterized as being something different from being nonserious. The mother had been presented with a choice: not serious/possibly serious. Depending on how the mother understood the doctor's use of the word "but", the gallery of routine was either maintained or thrown into question.

One way parents employed to get out of making the choice between one side or the other in a side-by-side was to draw a distinction which questioned the validity of the side-by-side frame itself. In Excerpt G, both the mother and father challenged the mother's presentation of the frames she had heard in the doctor's office. They both questioned the rims of the frames (Keeney, 1990a). Keeney, following Goffman (1974), described the rim of a frame as an indication of "how the content was to be taken, typically in terms of 'real' or 'fiction' " (p. 64). In Excerpt G, the parents suggested that the content of the frames might be highly questionable because the mother might have misinterpreted the doctor's talk about the heart murmur. If the rims throw doubt on their contents, then the information as presented by the mother could not challenge the routine gallery and the gallery was maintained.

The final transcription of the previous section (N) clearly illustrated how openings were created during the discovery/referral process. Keeney (1990a) stated that openings were frames in one gallery that provided doors, leaks, or transitions to new, different galleries. The discourse uttered in one gallery would be understood differently from those of the other gallery. In Excerpt N, the mother presented a series of frames which helped to maintain the routine gallery:

G1: Routine Medical Checkup
  F: "they ran an EKG"
  F: "some X rays"
  F: "she thought it [the murmur] looked fine"

Then the mother added another frame:

  F: "but she'd [the doctor] rather a cardiologist look at it"

The last frame was called an opening because it could have allowed the flow of discourse to follow a path which would have taken it out of the routine context/gallery. What did the phrase "but she'd rather a cardiologist look at it" mean? Did it mean that having a cardiologist was more of the same (i.e., routine) or did it mean that something was amiss with the process (i.e., not routine)? How was involving a cardiologist presented so that the gallery of routine could have been maintained, or how was referring to a pediatric cardiologist mentioned so as to provide a leak in a routine gallery? The same dilemma was also seen in the presentation of what was and was not a referable heart murmur.

REFERABLE HEART MURMURS

In this study, two different groups were identified: those families with prior knowledge that their child had a heart murmur and those who had no such awareness. But in either case, all the families were faced with a *new* perspective: Their child was now being diagnosed as having a *referable* heart murmur, a medical situation which required the expertise of a pediatric cardiologist. As shown above in Excerpt E, one family, who had come to see the doctor about their teenage son's bad knees, had known of their son's heart murmur since he was a small child, but their current physician now contextualized the old label (heart murmur) with a new set of procedures (referral to a pediatric cardiologist). This shift in how the child was being treated can be unsettling to the family: What is now known about the child's condition which mandates a visit to a heart specialist? In the interviews, family members expressed different ways in which learning of the referable heart murmur was discomforting.

For some families, the news of a referable heart murmur brought to light a contrast between the parents' observations of their child's seemingly healthy behavior and the label of referable heart murmur.

Excerpt O

(01) *M:* . . . even with Robert we haven't noticed anything wrong with
(02) him, he seems just as normal as any other kids. I sure don't stop
(03) him from jumping around and running around all day long.

In Excerpt O, the mother, after learning that her son had a heart murmur, voiced doubt about her and her husband's perception of their son's health: "he *seems* [italics added] just as normal as any other kids." In Excerpt P, the mother and father, whose son's diagnosis was changed from irregular heartbeat to heart murmur, had not thought much about their son's heart because he had always been quite active.

Excerpt P

(01) *M:* Okay. (.) And so I said you know we really didn't think much
(02) about because he's very active he's never tired unless (.)
(03) *F:* He's bored
(04) *M:* if he's bored, he's tired. You know and as long as he's having fun
(05) we know that he thinks about you know (.) hurting or anything
(06) like that or getting chest pains or anything like that. I didn't
(07) worry about it but and also I didn't worry about it because I had
(08) noticed that when they do a nose and (.) ear (.) check and throat
(09) *I:* Uh hum
(10) *M:* Uh they usually do an ((   )) pulse . . .

For most of the families in the study there were no observable physical abnormalities. This could have confused the families in light of what the physicians were now saying in regards to the children. Kreps and Thornton (1984, p. 100) referred to such situations in health communication as double-binds. Families were faced with a situation in which they needed to reconcile two seemingly contradictory positions: the doctor's diagnosis of a referable heart murmur and the family's observations of what they believed was a healthy child.

Another source of uneasiness for the family was the contradiction between referable and nonreferable heart murmurs. A nonreferable heart murmur was most likely one of the innocent variety (McNamara, 1987b) and one which should have caused little concern for the family. But what about a referable heart murmur? As stated earlier, a referable heart murmur could be a significant murmur, an indicator of serious heart problems (Paraskos, 1988). Such a heart murmur would be cause for alarm and worry on the part of the family.

In Excerpt Q, the mother not only expressed her worry over her child's condition, she also voiced her concern over which of the doctor's seemingly contradictory messages to follow: The doctor said not to worry and the doctor referred my child to a heart specialist. This left the mother with a variety of choices: (a) to worry over her child's condition, (b) not to worry over her child's condition, and (c) to worry over whether or not she should worry over her child's condition.

Excerpt Q

(01) *I:* But there's still a little bit of
(02) *M:* of doubt yeah (.)
(03) *I:* something
(04) *M:* cuz there there's a doubt in my mind (.) that it is (.) she [the
(05) doctor] wouldn't have it [referred my child] if there isn't anything
(06) wrong (.) so (.) I don't know I guess we'll find out today fer sure (.)
(07) *I:* Okay .hhh so even they say even though they said don't worry
(08) it's nothing serious it's (.)
(09) *M:* I worry
(10) *I:* why would they say it if
(11) *M:* right I worry
(12) *I:* There must be some reason there's a heart murmur you
(13) worry
(14) *M:* Mm hmm (.) right (.)

Excerpt R also clearly illustrated how families could react to the double-bind message that "the heart murmur was not serious, but your child should be sent to a heart specialist in order to be really sure." Both the father in Line 02 ("We didn't know what to think.") and the mother in Lines 08 and 09 ("So we didn't react.") expressed the paralyzing qualities of being caught in a double bind. Again, in Lines 05 through 09, the mother clearly expressed the oscillation that families might have gone through as they tried to decide which of the two contradictory messages they should follow: "We know that it's serious [It's a referable/noninnocent heart murmur.] but we didn't know how to react if it was a serious thing [It's a referable/noninnocent heart murmur.] or just you know like a functional murmur [It's a referable/innocent heart murmur.].

Excerpt R

(01) *I:* I can imagine how you felt, but can you say it too now you felt at
(02) the time?
(03) *F:* We didn't know what to think.
(04) *M:* I didn't (laughter)
(05) *F:* We didn't know how serious [it would be]
(06) *M:* We didn't know whether to take it seriously or (.) We know that
(07) its serious but we didn't know how to react if it if was a real
(08) serious thing or just you know like a functional murmur. So we
(09) don't didn't react. We were in a state of just there (laughter).
(10) *F:* (( )) see what happens.

In Excerpt S, the family expressed reactions similar to those stated by the parents in Excerpt R. When faced with the dilemma of how to feel about the referral, these families chose not to feel ("I don't know how to feel," "On hold," and ". . . numb"). The mother and the father in Excerpt S were able to delay the decision of whether to worry or not until they received more information because as the mother said, "Nothing you can do one way or the [other] just (.) live with it (laughter)."

Excerpt S

(01) *I:* How do you mean, haven't felt?
(02) *M:* I don't know how to feel, you know like I said earlier, I don't
(03) know how to feel about this. I'm just gonna take it as it goes, one
(04) day at a time.
(05) *I:* It's almost kind of, not even having enough information to know
(06) what to feel. So more . . . numb? Is that it, or on hold?
(07) *M:* On hold, yeah.
(08) *I:* Does that kind of fit for you too?
(09) *F:* I think so.
(10) *I:* Kind of on hold until you get some more answers.
(11) *F:* Yeah, I don't want to get (.) too excited, and it might not be
(12) nothing to get all excited about. (( )) Just stay cool.
(13) *M:* Nothing you can do one way or the [other] just (.) live with it
(14) (laughter).

But a referable heart murmur could also be an innocent heart murmur. The referring physician just wanted to confirm the diagnosis. The physician may not have had either the confidence, time, expertise, and/or equipment to make a definitive statement on the murmur; therefore, to be absolutely positive, a referral was made. For some families, there was a need to know more about the circumstance surrounding the referral. In Excerpt T, the mother attempted to elicit more of this type of information from the doctor and his staff.

Excerpt T

(01) *M:* I asked the receptionist and she said you know cause I asked her,
(02) "Is him sending him to Lubbock does it signify anything?" And
(03) she says "no not really, she said we really can't say anything
(04) until we get the results of the test."

As the mother recalled in Excerpt T, the receptionist's answer of "no not really" to the question whether the referral was worthy of worry was contradicted by her subsequent stating "we can't say anything until we get the results of the tests." If the doctor and staff could not say anything until they received the test results, how could they be sure that the referral did not signify anything to be worried about; the results could show that the murmur was significant.

Situations such as the one described above in Excerpt T, helped to create additional concerns on the parts of the parents: If the referring physician did not know enough to make the diagnosis himself or herself, did the referring physician know enough about what he or she does and does not know? Is it a question of whether or not general practitioners know what they don't know? If the families were in doubt about what the non-heart specialist knew about the heart, then the families might doubt the label of "innocent" for the heart murmur.

In Excerpt U, the mother and father discussed their interpretations of the referring doctors' diagnosis of their child's heart murmur. The parents had been concerned about the lack of information they had received from the physicians. At first, the couple considered that the doctors were withholding information—information that might have alarmed them. In Lines 11 and 12, the father offered an alternative understanding of the lack of information: "because I don't think they [the referring physicians] knew all that much about it [the heart murmur] (.)." It was not clear from the parents' conversation if their questioning of the doctors' knowledge caused them to doubt the validity of the referral or if the referral made perfect sense given the doctors' alleged ignorance of heart murmurs.

Excerpt U

(01) *I:* So it wasn't even clear answers saying I don't know but kind of
(02) *M:* right
(03) *I:* evasive or hedging or unclear
(04) *M:* just more like
(05) *F:* yes
(06) *M:* saying
(07) *F:* take her and get it checked out some more
(08) *I:* See someone else we did
(09) *F:* who knows more about her problem
(10) *I:* Mm Hmm
(11) *F:* because I don't think they [the referring physicians] knew all that
(12) much about it [the heart murmur] (.)

Families had certain expectations of what physicians should be able to do as far as providing medical services were concerned. Some families believed that doctors should be experts for all areas of the body. Of course, all physicians cannot be experts or specialists for all areas of medical concern. In the case of cardiological knowledge, it was not uncommon for families to expect that the primary care physician know as much about the heart as he or she knew about any other organ system (McNamara, 1987b). When a physician appeared to be hesitant or uncertain with a diagnosis, this might have suggested to the family that something was being held back from them or what was being said was not enough for the family to be satisfied.

Given their understanding that the doctor was supposed to know about their child's condition, the families in the next two excerpts (V and W) gave *accounts* (Scott & Lyman, 1968) for why the doctors were unable or unwilling to give parents their anticipated answers. Scott and Lyman (1968) described an account as "a statement made by a social actor to explain unanticipated or untoward behavior—whether that behavior is his [sic] own or that of others . . ." (p. 46). In the case for these families and others in this study, the untoward or unanticipated behavior was that of the expert (the doctor) not acting like an expert (not knowing all of the answers).

The family in Excerpt V gave an account for the doctor's hesitancy (Lines 10–11). The mother offered that the doctor might have tried to explain, but had been unsuccessful (Lines 07–08) and that telling the family certain information might not have been the doctor's place (Lines 15–17). Stokes and Hewitt (1976) also called these types of account-giving, *aligning actions:* "largely verbal efforts to restore or assure meaningful interaction in the face of problematic situations of one kind or another . . . , formulating the definition of a situation and talking about motives illustrate a dual process of alignment" (p. 838). In

Excerpt V, the father identified a problematic situation: "the questions that the doctor never told her [the man's wife] that (.) what could be done to help her [his daughter]. Later, the wife supplied possible motives why the doctor would have behaved in such a manner: maybe it was not the doctor's place to have told her the needed information (Lines 15–17).

Excerpt V

(01) *I:* Okay (.) has it been anyone who's made it hard or difficult (.) or
(02) confusing
(03) *M:* no not really (( ))
(04) *F:* Just the questions that the the doctor never told her [his wife]
(05) that (.) what could be really done to help her [his daughter]
(06)
(07) *M:* I mean I think that they should've (.) more of less tried to explain
(08) something to me
(09) *I:* So then not explaining made it more difficult
(10) *M:* I guess Doctor Flemons (.) may have tried but he was (.) hesitant
(11) for some reason (.) to me he was
(12) *I:* Okay
(13) *M:* for some reason he was
(14) *I:* (( )) to both of you okay
(15) *M:* ah huh (.) I don't know why but (.) I'm hoping it's not for any (.)
(16) I figure that he should've told me to begin with whether (.) it was
(17) his place or not (.)

In Excerpt W, the mother gave accounts for why she was unable to get information from her doctor: "he's strange," "he's always in a hurry," "He kinda talks funny," and "Yeah, kind of evasive." As was also seen in Excerpt V, when faced with a situation in which the expert (the doctor) did not have all the answers, these families attempted to supply excuses or accounts in order to help make sense of a problematic situation.

Excerpt W

(01) *M:* I really didn't have time to think about it. Cause I volunteered to
(02) work at the clinic that day, so I was busy . . .
(03) *I:* Oh, you were working . . .
(04) *M:* I was busy with other students.
(05) *I:* So probably as soon as you could you got out of there and said
(06) let's go check it out more.
(07) *M:* Yes. Exactly. (laughter)
(08) *I:* Did you ask him any other questions?
(09) *M:* Uh um. Nothing. Dr. Girardi is very (.) he's strange and he doesn't
(10) really, he's doesn't really he's always like in a hurry so you really

(11) don't have time to corner him (laughter) and ask him questions.
(12) *F:* He kinda talks funny, you got to really, he's one of (( ))
(13) *I:* (( ))
(14) *F:* ((Talks)) ((he's a pretty good doctor))
(15) *I:* But sometimes hard to get hold him down to get answers (( )).
(16) *F:* Yeah, kind of evasive (( )).

In Excerpt X, the mother expressed her concern about what the referring physicians might *not* know about her child; maybe there was something more to be known about the case and that new knowledge might have contradicted the innocent heart murmur label.

Excerpt X
(01) *I:* Did you ask them when you were with the other doctors
(02) *M:* I asked (.) well (what it is but) its like (.) they don't (.) its (.) well
(03) its not like they're giving you the runaround it's (.) I guess unless
(04) they don't know why it it does sound to me like they don't know
(05) *I:* like they don't know okay
(06) *M:* if they cuz if they knew they would have told me something and
(07) (.) you know (( ))

By not receiving the expected answers, the family members may have become frustrated with the physicians. As seen above (Excerpt X), the mother began to speculate possible reasons for the doctor's clinical uncertainty (Brenner, Ringel, & Berman, 1984). She was having trouble reconciling not hearing what she wanted to hear (i.e., definitive answers on her child's heart) and the fact that the doctor had earlier told her that there was nothing about which to worry. So when the general practitioner announced the decision of referral to the heart specialist by saying, "It's nothing to worry about," the families could still choose to be worried. They were able to question the non-heart expert's position on really knowing whether they should worry or not. In addition, the family members could have questioned the incongruity between the doctor's "not-to-worry" statements and the doctor's actions of referring the family to a specialist so as to be really sure.

Excerpt Y
(01) *I:* Anything about the experience that has tripped you up or
(02) frustrated you or anything like that?
(03) *M:* I guess I was concerned (.) I was hearing it was something he
(04) would grow out of and I guess maybe just thought of following
(05) up on it maybe it might be serious.
(06) *I:* So even though it was something that he would grow out of it (.)
(07) it was a developmental thing normal thing you still need to come
(08) in for an appointment . . .
(09) *M:* It was something you know why make an appointment if its
(10) normal (.) why not make it [the appointment] a year [from now]

The mother in Excerpt Y became concerned because not only was the doctor referring her child for "something he would grow out of," but this referral was one that could not wait ("why not make it [the appointment] a year [from now]"). Many families found the referral process ambiguous and, as seen above, "referral" could mean many different things. Barnlund (1984), when addressing ambiguity in medical settings had stated,

> If so many words are vague in their reference, messages composed of such ambiguous elements will be even less precise. Nearly every statement can support many legitimate and even contradictory interpretations. In some respects the vocabulary of illness constitutes a special case. (p. 45)

RFA of Referable Heart Murmurs

How a referable heart murmur was defined either maintained the gallery of routine/nonproblematic medical encounters or created openings to alternative galleries of nonroutine/problematic medical encounters for the families. At the center of the defining was the relationship between frames and events.

Keeney (1990a) outlined the different distinctions which were possible considering the relationship between frames and events. The possibilities were

Same Frame; Same Events
Different Frame; Same Events
Same Frame; Different Events
Different Frame; Different Events

Same Frame referred to the continuance of a context whereas Different Frame meant that there had been a recontextualization.

In connection to heart murmurs, Same Frame meant that the child's diagnosis remained unchanged through the process: The child had been previously diagnosed as having a heart murmur and that diagnosis was upheld by the referring physician. Of course, the opposite could also have been true: The child could have been previously diagnosed as *not* having a heart murmur and that diagnosis was also upheld. The involvement of such a child in this study was highly unlikely, but it could have occurred due to a miscommunication or mishearing (e.g., A family could have come to the pediatric cardiologist by mistake or the interviewers in the study could have mistakenly interviewed a family not designated for this study).

Different Frame meant that there was a difference between the diagnosis of heart murmur and how the families perceived their child's heart prior to the diagnosis. For instance, before the referral to the pediatric cardiologist, the family may have had no awareness of a heart murmur in their child or there could have been other heart diagnoses (e.g., irregular heartbeat). Different Frame could also have meant that there was a shift from a heart murmur diagnosis to no heart murmur in the diagnosis or to another heart diagnosis. These transforms will be the focus in a later section of this chapter.

The other side of the distinction, Events, referred to a change or stabilization of content in relation to the Same or Different Frames. Same Events in this study meant no change in treatment for the child (i.e., no referral of the child, no involvement of additional medical personnel, etc.). Different Events was taken to mean that a change in treatment had occurred (i.e., the child had been referred to a pediatric cardiologist). All of the families in the study would have fallen under this last distinction. The point of making this distinction was that it was based on observable behavior and not on semantics. In other words, the act of the family coming to the hospital was taken to be Different Events, whether or not the families considered this to be a change for them. This was done in order to investigate variations in how the families contextualized their visit. They could have negated the Different Events label or they could have described the meaning of the label, but the focus of the study was on the coming to the hospital.

Given the two sides of the relationship (Frame/Events), and given the two distinctions on each side (Same/Different), there were four groups possible, but only two were likely to be represented in this study due to the restriction that the sample was to be composed of *only* children with

Same Frame	/	*Different Events*
Prior Heart Murmur Diagnosis	/	Referral to Pediatric Cardiologist

and

Different Frame	/	*Different Events*
No Prior Knowledge of Child's Heart Murmur	/	Referral to Pediatric Cardiologist

For the Same Frame / Different Events group, there was a change in treatment (referral) and for the Different Frame/ Different Events groups, there were two changes: a change in diagnosis and a change in treatment. It could be argued that there were two changes for both groups because the change in events (referral) could have recontextualized the original heart murmur diagnosis

F: Referable
  f: heart murmur

if the act of referral was taken to mean something different for the family (i.e., nonroutine). That was the main question or concern of this study: "How would the referral to a pediatric cardiologist be contextualized by the family?" The question was extremely important when the larger context of routine/nonroutine was considered. If the gallery of routine medical encounters (G1) was not maintained, then what would be the repercussions in the larger context? G1 was most likely embedded in a larger gallery of a healthy child (G0). Depending on how the referral was handled, the gallery of

G0: Healthy child
G1: Routine Check up
    F: Routine referral

healthy child would have been maintained or it would have leaked.

G0: Healthy child
G1: Routine checkup
    F: Routine referral / Nonroutine referral

Excerpts O and P were good examples of how families began to question the fit between the gallery of healthy child with the frame of referral: "even with Robert we haven't noticed anything wrong with him, he seems just as normal as any other kids" (O) and "he's very active he's never tired unless—he's bored" (P). Some families had to struggle with what they saw as contradictory frames: healthy child/referable heart murmur.

The struggle came from the ambiguity of what was a referable heart murmur: was there a referral to confirm innocence or a referral to confirm significance?

F: Referable Heart Murmur? (A little doubt)

f: innocent	f: significant
They said it's not serious	She wouldn't have referred it if?

In contrast to the family in O were the mother and father in Excerpt R. When faced with the choice between innocent and significant, they made the choice of not making the choice: "So we didn't react." The same phenomenon was seen in Excerpt S: "Nothing you can do one way or the [other] just (.) live with it (laughter).

Another dilemma faced by families who strived to end the oscillation was the referring physician's ability to know what he or she did and did not know. It was another rim-of-the-frame situation: Was the doctor a heart expert and therefore the diagnosis was unquestionable or was the doctor a nonheart expert and therefore the diagnosis was questionable?

In the previous situation, both frames were the same, but the meanings were very different.

Rim: Doctor as expert	Rim: Doctor as nonexpert
F: Innocent heart murmur	F: Innocent heart murmur

It was also a question of fit for the mother in Excerpt Y:

Rim: Expert /Nonexpert

F:	Something he would grow out of just follow up on it	/	F: It was something you know why make an appointment if it's normal (.) why not make it [the appointment] a year [from now]

The mother felt that there was an incongruity between a frame of *it's normal* and another frame *make an appointment now*. For many parents, the lack of fit between frames lead them to try to make sense of the difference they perceived between the frame of the murmur as *not being serious* and the frame of the murmur *needs to be heard by a cardiologist*. Two ways in which families went about dealing with this problem were to transform the meaning of the heart murmur and to seek out alternative sources of information.

TRANSFORMS

Faced with such dilemmas of interpretation, what choices have families had in attempting to understand seemingly ambiguous messages? One possibility was to transform either the act of referral or the label of heart murmur into more serious acts and/or labels. Families might have created a series of "what if's" in response to hearing that their child had a referable heart murmur. For example, in the two following transcriptions (Z and AA), one mother feared that the next logical step in the referral process could have been surgery for her child and another mother expressed concern about what it would mean if the pediatric cardiologist had to ask the family to come back to the hospital again.

Excerpt Z

(01) *I:* So you're afraid not only about the surgery, but also like what if
(02) something more happened.
(03) *M:* Yeah, (.) yeah.

Excerpt AA
(01) *M:* We don't wanna have to come back again (.) cuz I know he if we
(02) come back again it's just gonna mean that they're gonna have to
(03) do something different

The following excerpt (BB) illustrated how one mother transformed the meaning of what a referable heart murmur was for her. The decision to see the heart specialist was decided because "it was something that couldn't wait your heart is the only thing that keeps you going."

Excerpt BB
(01) *I:* . . . what kinds of things went into the decision to go ahead and
(02) make the appointment to come here
(03) *M:* I felt like it was something that couldn't wait your heart is the
(04) only thing that keeps you going I wanted to get it done before
(05) school started and wanted to know how bad it was

As stated earlier, a referral which focused on an individual's heart could cause concern (Hersher, 1988). The ambiguous nature of heart murmurs was such that it was quite normal for families to associate an innocent heart murmur with either a significant heart murmur, heart disease, or even death (Bergman & Stamm, 1967; Hersher, 1988). The pathologizing of a benign condition such as an innocent heart murmur helped to create what Meador (1965) termed as nondisease. A nondisease occurred when individuals acted as if they had a condition which should have been treated as a disease when in reality they did not have that disease. Bergman and Stamm (1967) warned that when families were referred for innocent heart murmurs there should be an "appreciation of the morbidity possible in cardiac nondisease" (p. 1012). Families whose children did not have heart disease might have begun to treat their child as if he or she had a disease as a result of the diagnosis of an innocent heart murmur.

One possible indication of parents' perceiving that their child was vulnerable is that they would begin to treat their child as if he or she really did have a serious heart condition (e.g., special treatment at home). As seen in the next passage (CC), a mother recalled how a referring physician had to work very hard in order to stave off the parent's attempts to seek permission to treat her child as if the diagnosis was something more serious than a heart murmur.

Excerpt CC
(01) *M:* Yeah (.) and I'd ask Dr. Benjamin if I needed to treat him
(02) different, I mean do something different. When she first told us in
(03) the hospital, cause I went home before he was even 24 hours old.

> I said "Do you think we should stay here." "No, there's no need to stay." And then in her office I asked her again well, "Should I do anything ah different?" And by that I meant you know like keep him away (from) people, was what I was getting at. "Not here's nothing different to do." And she explained that one's that had real bad heart murmurs, looks different, and she could feel the heart murmur from outside the chest. She gave us several different symptoms all of which she said he didn't have. She said "we wouldn't even know he had [one], if we didn't have the stethoscope to hear it." So that that part helped, when she explained it that way.

RFA of Transforms

Within the gallery of healthy child, some parents began to transform the meaning of innocent heart murmur into something much more severe (for example, significant heart murmur, heart disease, death). This process of transforming, in some cases, helped to shift parents' discourse from a gallery of healthy child to a gallery of unhealthy child.

The beginnings of this transforming process were found in the initial side-by-side distinction set up with the dilemma of what was a referable heart murmur:

F: innocent   F: significant
    f: heart murmur   f: heart murmur
F: referable heart murmur
    f: innocent   f: significant

The basic distinction was between the absence of pathology (innocent) and the presence of pathology (significant). Many parents kept oscillating between the two sides of the same distinction, but some transformed one type or class of the nonpathology/pathology distinction (innocent/significant) to another class of the same basic nonpathology/pathology distinction.

nonpathology	/	pathology
F: innocent	/	F: significant
F: heart nondisease	/	F: heart disease
F: life	/	F: death

Significance, heart disease, and death were all on the same side of the nonpathology/pathology distinction but were all in different classes. Transforming a significant heart murmur to heart disease was a simple manner as parents followed the nonpathology/pathology to a logical conclusion. As the talk shifted to the graver classes of this distinction, the gallery of healthy child was also transformed to a gallery of unhealthy child. This was what Bergman and Stamm (1967) and Hersher (1988) warned about when they cited the vulnerable child literature (Green & Solnit, 1964) as having relevance with referable heart murmurs.

The recursive nature of frame and content of frame would be such that something like a *vicious circle* (Watzlawick, 1984) would be created. Watzlawick descibed the phenomenon of a vicious circle as

> the sequence of events which was not rectilinear, but in which the effect fed back upon its own cause. This happened in nearly every marital conflict that turned and turned on itself in the same vicious manner, whose starting point was beyond recall and, even if recalled, no longer matters. (p. 65)

Watzlawick went on to say that the notion of the vicious circle was similar to the how Heinz von Foerster (1984a) defined cognition (i.e., "computations of computations of computations . . . p. 48), and that "once established, such a circle was beyond beginning and end, and beyond cause and effect" (p. 65). The healthy child context/healthy child discourse shifted to unhealthy child context/unhealthy child discourse, and this oscillation (healthy to unhealthy) could have continued until some sort of intervention could have been made which might have been able to disrupt the cycle.

Excerpt CC was a good example of how the parents' talk was clearly in the gallery of unhealthy child and how the doctor created opening or leaks in that gallery which allowed the mother to leave the unhealthy child gallery and return to the gallery of the healthy child.

G: Unhealthy Child
- F: I'd ask Dr. Benjamin if I needed to *treat him different, I mean do something different* (mother)
  - f: Should we stay her [in the hospital] (mother)
    - f: No, there's no need to stay (Doctor) - LEAK
- F: Should I do anything different?
  - f: Keep him away (from) people
  - f: No - real bad heart murmurs, looks different - LEAK
  - f: She could feel [a real bad heart murmur] - LEAK
  - f: symptoms he didn't have - LEAK

So that part help, when she explained it [the innocent heart murmur] that way [The murmur was not significant.] - GALLERY EXIT to Gallery of Healthy Child

The doctor in Excerpt CC presented frames which helped to switch the talk from a gallery which focused on the pathology side of the distinction to one on the nonpathology side. Another way to describe what the doctor did was to say that she was involved in the process of frame destruction (Keeney, in press): the deliberate eradication of a context. (In this case, the context was that of an unhealthy child,) If the doctor was unable to turn the flow of talk over to the nonpathology side, the rest of the referral process might have been understood by the parent as being in a context or gallery of an unhealthy child.

It would be unwise to think that this would be the last time that this or any parent would question the healthy child/unhealthy child distinction during the referral process. There were many potential leaks and opening in the families' discourse ecology that would threaten the maintenance of the healthy child as the families continued to interact with each other. In addition, parents talked with other people, read articles, or consulted with medical books. All of these alternative sources of information were potential leaks and potential maintainers to the families' galleries.

ALTERNATIVE SOURCES OF INFORMATION

Another reaction families had after hearing that their child had a referable heart murmur was to seek out corroborating evidence that would help them decide how to contextualize the medical news they had heard from the referring physician. An obvious choice was for families to go seek out other primary care physicians before seeing the pediatric cardiologist and this was done by a few of families in this study.

Besides other physicians, families also went to other available health care professionals for facts. The mother in the next segment (DD) worked at a hospital and was able to go to nurses with whom she worked. The nurses provided the mother with additional and possibly contradictory information from what the doctor had told the mother.

Excerpt DD

(01) *M:* And uh, uh I asked what it was. See I work I'm a nurse's aide
(02) and I work at Greenfield Hospital and I asked a few nurses and
(03) they said a heart murmur and they told me that the heart was
(04) weak.

Some families sought out additional information from medical books and reference materials. The mother in Excerpt EE referred to a book she had on childhood diseases. The book could have been any one of a number of popular reference books on family health and care, [e.g., *The American Medical Association Family Medical Guide* (Kunz & Finkel, 1987); *Better Homes and Gardens New Family Medical Guide* (Kiester, Jr., 1982); *Good Housekeeping Family Health & Medical Guide* (1979)], available in most libraries or bookstores. The mother, having recalled reading that "50% of all children under 13 or something had heart murmurs at some time," seemed to be able to contextualize her child's heart murmur as not being so worrisome.

Excerpt EE

M: We talked to your parents, anybody, family, friends. Have they been supportive, helpful in this?

I: So rather than saying, "I don't know, I don't know, I don't know." Wait till you . . .

M: Right. Yeah. Cause you know people are concerned and they don't. They'd probably ask me stuff and just upset me, or tell me stories. So we just don't say anything (( ))

I: So really wanting to hear it from the expert, from Dr. Smith, what she has to say.

M: Right. Yeah. And it helped (( )) doctor when home and pulled out my book, you know on childhood diseases, you know.

I: Um hmm

M: Cause that helped some. You know, and it was saying 50% of all children under 13 or something had heart murmurs at some time. But you know I still don't understand what kind it was cause you know it talked about the ones like my daughter had that are acquired or whatever

I: Um hmm

M: And then the ones that are congenital. And I understand what I was reading (( ))

In contrast to the effects reading additional material had on the mother in excerpt EE was the reaction that the father in the next transcription (FF) had to reading a pamphlet on heart murmurs. While waiting in an office prior to being interviewed for this study, the father picked up a leaflet which discussed heart murmurs, both innocent and significant. Until reading this material, the father had not been worried about his daughter's heart murmur. He had had a heart murmur when he was a child and there had not been any serious complications for him resulting from having had a heart murmur as a child. But when reading the pamphlet, he discovered that some heart conditions associated with (significant) heart murmurs had to be corrected by heart surgery. This information provided the father with another prognosis for having a heart murmur, one which he had not considered before and one which caused him alarm.

Excerpt FF
(01) *F:* Yes but you know me having one and growing up with it (.) no
(02) I'm not worried too much until I read that pamphlet
(03) *I:* Okay so this is what scared you the most right now the pamphlet
(04) *F:* The pamphlet what's bothering me what's it stating

McNamara (1987a, 1987b, 1988) had recommended that families be given written material by the referring physician to help the parents and/or patient better understand the heart murmur diagnosis and referral. Being able to take a handout home would enable parents to have the physician's words at their disposal in case any scares, like the one mentioned above, occurred. If the parents heard or read any information on heart murmurs that might have led them to understand that their child's innocent heart murmur was significant in any way, all the parents would have to do was read over the doctor's expert opinion on murmurs and the crisis would be eliminated.

In addition to seeking out facts from other doctors, medical personnel, and reference books, families went to other, nonmedical sources in attempts to find expert information that would provide definitive answers for them. One popular source for material was friends and neighbors. In some cases, these nonmedical sources provided examples and anecdotes which put families at ease. The following quote (GG) showed how learning about the seriousness of a friend's child's heart condition helped one mother put her child's heart murmur into perspective.

Excerpt GG
(01) *M:* . . . Well, we also have some good friends that just had a baby
(02) with some real serious heart problems. So you know this is
(03) nothing. (laughter)

For another family, consultation with other sources only clouded the issue more. In the next transcription (HH), the good news of one neighbor was counterbalanced by two not as favorable reports from some other friends.

Excerpt HH
(01) *M:* Not really because they contradict each other. Some, my neighbor,
(02) her his little child it's the same age as his she's the same age as
(03) Roman and she was born with one but hers went away and she
(04) say's he say's "Oh it's nothing, he'll outgrow it." And then my
(05) other friend, she says, "Well, my cousin had one, but he had
(06) surgery and then some other one, an aunt I think she said . . . "
(07) *I:* This is (( ))
(08) *M:* Just a friend of mine.
(09) *I:* Oh.

(10) *M:* That hers was controlled with medication
(11) *I:* Oh her cousin.
(12) *I:* Um hum.
(13) *M:* You know so it's they contradict each other.
(14) *I:* So you don't know who to believe. Or they're both right, but it
(15) doesn't help you.

Besides consulting with friends, the parents also drew upon their own family history for information. Some families had considerable experience with heart problems in their families and even in their own lives. Again, as with the information from the friends and neighbors, the familial knowledge could have been contradictory: One relative had good results with heart problems while another relative died due to heart-related matters. For example, in the next two transcriptions, the mother in Excerpt II found her positive outcome with her own heart murmur to be a valuable resource for her during the referral process, while the mother in Excerpt JJ, even after hearing positive information from her own mother, still needed to wait for word from the doctor before she could stop worrying.

Excerpt II
(01) *M:* Really, (.) at this stage, until they tell me that something is wrong
(02) and that there's something serious that needs to be done, it's
(03) because of because what I went through, and because of what I
(04) remember of having a heart murmur, to me it's not any big deal.
(05) Simply because, it never nothing ever came of it. So if they tell
(06) me something's going on and we need to treat it, then we'll take
(07) it a little more seriously and do something about it, but until that
(08) I don't see any point in worrying about. You know, cause they
(09) just found it, and it's not something that, at this stage, hopefully,
(10) nothing harmful. So (( )) [work with that].

Excerpt JJ
(01) *M:* My mother. And she [her mother] told me something like that in
(02) lots of cases [the heart murmur] just naturally goes away as the
(03) child grows, so I don't know anything about it is, I just ah, wait
(04) for ever the doctor says.

One negative consequence of this searching for answers in their families' medical history had was that parents sometimes tended to blame themselves for their child's heart murmur. Maybe one side of the family had all the heart problems whereas the other side had no such occurrences. Besides blaming heredity, some parents began to reexamine their prenatal activities for possible causes of the heart murmur. Both of the mothers in the following two segments (KK and LL) alluded to medication they had taken during their pregnancies as having had some connection with their child's heart murmur.

Excerpt KK
(01) *M:* And one thing that really concerned me was some medication I
(02) had taken while I was pregnant for my for my headaches.
(03) *I:* Did that maybe uh
(04) *M:* Right that that might have had an effect on him. Yeah. That was
(05) my first thought (.) when they told me the heart murmur, that it
(06) was my fault.

Excerpt LL
(01) *M:* Uh. I was taking nerve medicine when I had when I was carrying
(02) him. So I was wondering if that had any effect.

For some families the innocent heart murmur diagnosis and referral brought a series of worries and concerns. There was doubt on some of the families' part as to why they were being sent to pediatric cardiologists. There were also definite concerns as to the vulnerability of their children. All of these concerns might have contextualized some parents' expectations of the consult with the heart specialist.

RFA of Alternative Sources For Information

The search for information that would have helped families to make a decision as to whether or not their child's heart murmur was significant or not was a good example of the difference between quantity and pattern (Bateson, 1979). If the process of gaining corroborating evidence was governed by notions of quantity, then it would have been a simple matter to decide the nature of the heart murmur: Add up the evidence and see which side had more and that would be the side of the distinction with which the family would have gone. But, in some instances, it only took a couple or even one noncorroborating frame to cause the healthy child/innocent heart murmur relationship to be shaken.

In Excerpt FF, the father had had a heart murmur. His sister had also had one. There were no examples in his familial background that would have prescribed a flip to the pathology side of the distinction. All of this was changed by his reading of a pamphlet in the doctor's office. The information in the pamphlet did not fit with the context he had constructed. It provided the father with a new lens or frame which helped him to create an alternative view of his child's heart murmur (Keeney, 1983). The change of frame or rather the change in the relationship between frame and content had made a difference which made a difference for the father: The father now had a frame of significant heart murmur with which to view the discovery/referral process. Although there was a significant amount of evidence on the nonpathology side, the pattern of frame to content was changed by a single frame which did not fit the previous pattern. This was an important point.

As was stated above, for some families the search for more, or rather, different information was a precarious process. Parents searched for frames which would have helped them out of the contexts of indecision and ambiguity. For the mother in Excerpt GG, the news of her friend's baby's heart difficulties helped her to contextualize her own child's heart situation as being nothing serious:

F1: Nonpathology/pathology ambiguity of own child
  f: Friend's baby's "real serious problems"
F2: Nonpathology of own child—"So you know that this is nothing serious (laughter)"

The process was similar for those families who searched their own family history in order to alleviate the referable heart murmur ambiguity. One interesting side effect of this search occurred when the talk about the child shifted to the gallery of unhealthy child. Within that gallery, one logical and predictable pattern was for parents to construct causes for the heart murmur. This was another example of what Bergman and Stamm (1967) meant when they cited Meador's (1965) nondisease phenomena. The innocent heart murmur frame was now in the gallery of unhealthy child, and with the shift to a disease orientation, parents naturally attempted to find causes, and in some instances, to lay blame for the heart murmur. Both excerpts KK and LL were examples of this type of talk:

RFA of Excerpt KK
  G: Unhealthy child
    F: Significant heart murmur
      f: ". . . some medication I had taken while I was pregnant for my headaches"
      f: "That was my first thought (.) when they told me the heart murmur, that it was my fault."
and RFA of Excerpt LL
  G: Unhealthy child
    F: Significant heart murmur
      f: "I was taking nerve medicine when I had when I carrying him."
      f: "So I was wondering if that had had any effect."

If these utterances were spoken in a gallery of healthy child, then the gravity of the prenatal activities would have been reduced: The heart murmur would have been inconsequential. If the talk was in the gallery of unhealthy child, and the discourse remains in that gallery, even if the medical consult with the specialist does not support the unhealthy child context, there could be some serious problems in the family. Would the parent and the child ever be able to leave the unhealthy/vulnerable child gallery?

The discovery/referral process was laden with many potential problems which would have to be dealt with by the family and the medical system, the referring physician and pediatric cardiologist. Depending on the pattern of leaks and gallery maintenance, the expectation of the parents and the delivery of information by the heart specialist would have produced different patterns.

EXPECTATIONS

For some families, the meaning of the innocent heart murmur had become unclear or remained ambiguous. The nature of what was and what was not a referable heart murmur had clouded the issue for a portion of the families. It was now up to the heart specialist to answer all the questions, to remove all of the doubts, and to clear up the ambiguities associated with referable heart murmurs. Bergman and Stamm (1967) characterized the demystification of heart murmurs as " 'delabeling' children" and wrote that delabeling was "one of the most frequently performed tasks of most pediatric cardiologists" (p. 1008).

Although delabeling was a commonplace occurrence for the cardiologist, it was a new, and sometimes frightening, experience for the parents. Although the mother in the next segment (MM) admitted that there were other serious worries in her life at that time, coming to the hospital to see the specialist had also been a concern for her.

Excerpt MM

(01) *I:* Sharon, what are your expectations for this examination (.) what
(02) are your expectations at this point?
(03) *M:* I'm really upset, I'd be lying if I was not (.)
(04) *I:* You're upset about? (.)
(05) *M:* This is something (.) that (.) and I'm probably stressed out
(06) anyway (.) now is a kinda hectic time in our lives (.) school, we
(07) just bought a house, and we hear about him (.) and they're trying
(08) to reduce my cortisone, my medication and this is not period
(09) now where I'm (.) full-blown (.) with this Lupus (.) my disease,
(10) and stress (.)
(11) *I:* So this is just a bad time (.)

For other families, their expectations were focused on receiving answers from the experts. Earlier in the interview, the mother in Excerpt NN had questioned the referring physician's knowledge of the heart (see Excerpt X). Now, she was anticipating the opportunity to hear from someone who would have medical acumen.

Excerpt NN

(01) *I:* Be up front up front with you and
(02) *M:* Right
(03) *I:* from the very beginning
(04) *M:* I think that's doctors are (.) are supposed to do
(05) *I:* Mm hmm
(06) *M:* Whether they're heart specialists or not (.)
(07) *I:* Mm hmm
(08) *M:* I think they should if if if they're I'm hopeful we're hopeful that
(09) it's that if there was anything that they're (.) that should've been
(10) (.) said to us (.) they should've told us
(11) *I:* Mm hmm
(12) *M:* He [the first referring physician] didn't and neither did Doctor
(13) Carlisle [the second referring physician] (.) we have to come all
(14) the way down here which is it's it's fine with us because seeing a
(15) heart specialist is just fine
(16) *I:* Mm hmm
(17) *M:* He'll know more about it and we wouldn't have to come down
(18) here
(19) *I:* So here today you get the answers (.)
(20) *M:* Yes

The same mother went on to state (Excerpt OO) that her confidence was not only based upon the specialist's knowledge of the heart ("there's doctors that know about the heart and other things"), but also upon the understanding that the cardiologist had the ability to know what she did and did not know about the heart ("I guess if she knows what she's talkin about well I can trust her").

Excerpt OO

(01) *M:* But if she [the pediatric cardiologist] knows (.) there's doctors that
(02) know about the heart and other things and I guess if she knows
(03) what she's talkin about well the I think I can trust her

Another expectation a few families had was the worry that the heart specialist would not be able to clear up the ambiguity of the referable heart murmur, or worse, that the cardiologist would discover that the child's condition was graver than had been anticipated by the family. For the family in the next transcription (PP), the concern for bad news and/or complications was quite present.

Excerpt PP

(01) *M:* Mm hmm so pretty good uh it's far it's been pretty good now it's
(02) just waiting for for the doctor we're hoping that it's nothing bad
(03) *I:* Sure
(04) *M:* We don't wanna have to come back again (.) cuz I know he if we
(05) come back again it's just gonna mean that they're [the pediatric
(06) cardiologists] gonna have to do something different

As has been seen, many families became quite concerned over the news of the referable heart murmur. They sought second opinions from a variety of sources, they questioned their activities during their pregnancies, and they pondered some life and death issues as a result of the referral to a pediatric cardiologist. But in contrast to these responses, there were some other instances during the interviews when families demonstrated how they handled the referral without becoming overly concerned and worried. They were able to contextualize the referral in such a way as to minimize their concerns.

RFA of Expectations

Parents' expectations were dominated by the talk that the pediatric cardiologist would be able to clear up the nonpathology/pathology ambiguity surrounding their child's referable heart murmur. What Bergman and Stamm (1967) called delabeling and RFA would call frame clearing (Keeney, 1990a) what was the parents anticipated from the heart specialists.

For some families, there was great confidence that the specialist would be able to cast all doubts aside because the cardiologist was clearly being identified as the expert on these matters of the heart. As was discussed in the RFA of Referable Heart Murmurs section, the rim of the frame was important in how families interpreted medical news from nonheart specialists: If the rim of the frame was questioned, so too would the content of threat frame. But, with the heart specialist, the rim was that of the expert: "He'll know more about it" (Excerpt NN) and "There's doctors that know about the heart . . ." (Excerpt OO).

One concern with frame clearing was that nonpathology frames could also have been cleared. The gallery of healthy child had been co-constructed by the parents and the non-heart specialists. What would happen if the heart specialist presented frames which did not fit within the healthy child gallery? This type of concern was quite present with some families:

Excerpt PP
G: Healthy child
F: "it's been pretty good not it's just waiting for the doctor
F: we're hoping that it's nothing bad (Clearing pathology frames)
F: We don't wanna come back (If nonpathology frame is cleared)
f: it's just gonna mean that they're gonna have to do thing different"

Other families were able to discuss their expectations of seeing the expert without mentioning concerns or worries that nonpathology frames could be cleared by the heart specialist. These families, for the most part, were able to take a wait-and-see attitude before making decisions to worry or not.

THE CHOICE NOT TO WORRY

In comparison to the times when families discussed their worries at length, there were other occasions when families did not seem to be upset about being referred to a pediatric cardiologist.

For example, the family in the next segment (QQ) had an interesting way of treating the news of a possible heart murmur. Their son had had numerous problems with his leg and so coming to see another specialist, albeit a heart specialist, was considered to be more of the same for them.

Excerpt QQ
(01) *M:* But we've been through years with him and we've been through
(02) his leg he had problems (.) So, it's not you know, we're just kinda
(03) like this is another (laughter).

For families like the one in the next excerpt (RR), the information as explained by the referring physician was enough for them to follow through with the referral without becoming too worried. They did not seem to focus in on the possible symbolic meaning of the referral, but instead, kept to the information provided by the primary care doctor.

Excerpt RR
(01) *M:* . . . because we have had something to base it on instead of just
(02) heart murmurs there's something, and Dr. Blake had even said to
(03) me, "Its just, I hear something there, it may be something he'll
(04) outgrow. I just want it checked out." So you know even from
(05) that, it's not a big concern, he just wants it checked.

For other families, there seemed to be a wait and see attitude: any decision to worry would hinge on the word of the expert—the heart specialist. They came to see the pediatric cardiologist to get the matter cleared up, but it was not apparent that they had bought into the referable heart murmur diagnosis of the referring physician.

The mother in the next transcription (SS) questioned the ability of the nurse who had first noticed the child's heart murmur. She seemed to be waiting for an expert's opinion before she decided to worry or not.

Excerpt SS

(01) *M:* It takes a medical doctor to see, to tell you if something is wrong
(02) with him, cause that is part of the work he does, cause he's all
(03) right. We're really hoping that maybe that nurse that checked him
(04) out was wrong about it.

For the mother in the following excerpt (TT), there appeared to be some concern that she did not have enough information in order to make a decision. Although she stated that she was scared when the doctor talked to her about her child's heart, she still could not recall or understand much of what was said to her prior to coming to see the cardiologist. It was unclear whether she was worried about her child's heart or whether she was worried that she did not have sufficient knowledge of the situation in order to judge the seriousness of the situation.

Excerpt TT

(01) *M:* Yeah, he (( )) the doctor scared me when he was talking about
(02) her heart.
(03) *I:* Do you remember what kinds of things he said that scared you?
(04) *M:* No. Not really. I forgot it.
(05) *I:* Maybe the way he talked or?
(06) *M:* Yeah, well I couldn't understand him much.
(07) *I:* Oh.
(08) *M:* Cause he has an accent.

The mother in the next example (VV) was worried about her child's health, but it was not necessarily because of the heart murmur diagnosis. She had been to another physician before seeing the doctor who successfully referred her to the pediatric cardiologist. Although she had heard about the murmur from the first physician who had referred her, she seemed to have delayed seeing a heart specialist because she felt that what the doctors were diagnosing as a heart murmur was really attributable to other illnesses from which her daughter was suffering at the time.

Excerpt VV

(01) *M:* . . . she had gone in for allergies. She was sick, she had sore
(02) throat and stuff. And then uh they I went back for her uh you
(03) know checkup on her, see how she was doing. And the doctor
(04) told me that they had heard a murmur in her heart. And I said no
(05) that was the first time and so they set me an appointment for the
(06) twenty-ninth of June and I didn't make it.

Yet, other families held off worrying because they were waiting for the heart expert to diagnose their child before they decided to worry. They came to the pediatric cardiologist in order to hear whether the referable heart murmur was innocent or significant (i.e., to have the cardiologist delabel the referable heart murmur). The families in this study expressed their desire to hear from the expert and that upon hearing the expert's diagnosis, then the families' worries would hopefully be over.

Excerpt VV

(01) *M:* But if she knows (.) there's doctors that know about the heart and
(02) other things and I guess if she knows talkin about well then I
(03) think I can trust her

And even if the news was not to be all good, then at least the family knew it was a definitive answer and they would be sure that there was cause for concern:

Excerpt WW

(01) *M:* So you know we're kind of just real open about it. And if there's
(02) a problem, and the doctors say, "We need to do something about
(03) this now," we'll do it. But until that point we're not going to be
(04) real anxious about it.

RFA of The Choice Not To Worry

Just as ambiguity and indecision made sense for some families in the study, clarity and decisiveness was the presiding logic for other parents. This latter group seemed to be able to keep their talk about their child's heart murmur in the gallery of healthy child. In Excerpt QQ, the family equated the heart murmur with a leg problem the child had had previously. The heart murmur was of a different class of medical problem, but it was understood as being in the nonpathology side as the leg problem which was cured:

nonpathology	/	pathology
previous leg problem	/	
current heart problem	/	

The key point was that the talk for this family remained entrenched in the healthy child gallery. One was the healthy child gallery was maintained was that the referral to the pediatric cardiologist was framed as being part of routine medical procedures. The referral, framed as routine, was not worrisome for parents and wold not have created a leak in the healthy child gallery. Excerpt RR was a good example of this logic:

G: Healthy child
  F: Routine check up / Routine Referral
    f: " 'It's just, I heart something there, it may be something he'll outgrow. I just want it checked out.' So you know even from that, it's not a big concern, he just wants it checked."

The mother's framing of the referral as not being a big concern confirmed and was confirmed by the healthy child gallery. For this family, referral to a pediatric cardiologist had a fit in the routine check up frame and in the larger healthy child gallery. The referral was not discussed as being a leak. It maintained and was maintained by the prevailing talk of the child as a healthy person.

Another way families kept from shifting into a pathology view of the heart was to set up a side-by-side distinction which threw doubt on the doctor's selection of the heart as being the cause of the child's ill health. The mother in Excerpt VV did not avoid the unhealthy child gallery, but she did create a distinction which helped her to doubt whether the child was ill due to a bad heart or whether the child's illness was attributable to other conditions:

G: Unhealthy child	/	A child with ill health
F: "a murmur in her heart"	or	F: She was sick, she had a sore throat

Her child was in ill health (sick) but not an unhealthy child (a bad heart). Whether or not the mother was clinically incorrect, her creation of alternative talk helped her avoid being overly concerned such that she was able to delay seeing the cardiologist the first time she had been referred.

Another way in which families were able to stay out of the oscillation between pathology/nonpathology was to decide to postpone making a decision until the expert had spoken. It was as if the families had set aside a blank frame, a frame whose content could only be filled by the expert—a pediatric cardiologist. The not-hearing of the expert's diagnosis was tolerable to these families because the blank or deciding frame remained within the gallery of healthy child. This concept was similar to what Bateson (1979) discussed when he wrote:

> in the circumstance that zero, the complete absence of any indicative event, can be a message. . . . The letter that you do not write, the apology you do not offer, the food that you do not put out for the cat—all these can be sufficient and effective messages because zero, *in context*, [emphasis from original source] can be meaningful; and *it is the recipient of the message who creates the context* [italics added]. (p. 51)

To these families, no message was confirmation of a healthy child and they would wait until the pediatric cardiologist supplied them with the definitive confirmation of the lack of a serious heart condition. To paraphrase a rather well-known legal dictum, The heart murmur was innocent until proven serious.

CONCLUSION

This chapter examined the talk of the families about the experiences surrounding their child's referral for a heart murmur. A few basic distinctions were drawn through the use of Recursive Frame Analysis. RFA allowed for a description of the talk which helped to make the flow of discourse understandable. What was not done in this chapter was to use these basic distinctions to help prescribe ways in which discourse could be managed such that families and medical personnel could be helped through the discovery/referral process. Chapter 5 attempts to present ways in which frame management can be applied to this process.

Chapter 5
Prescriptions, Implications, and Conclusions

INTRODUCTION

Although it is simple to describe families' interpretations of the referral process, it is quite another matter to prescribe to doctors and other medical personnel what they should and should not do as they refer families to specialists in the future. The issue of researcher as prescriptivist (Fairman, 1989) is not one to be taken lightly: The position of one discipline (systemic therapy/sociolinguistics) recommending, even suggesting, how another discipline (medicine) carries out its affairs can suggest a hierarchical relationship between the two disciplines.

Currently, there is a similar debate in linguistics as to the rules by which the linguist should act as an investigator. Fairman (1989, p. 3) argues that "students of modern linguistics are taught that the first task of a linguist is to describe how languages are used, not to prescribe how they should be used." He also warns against prescription which disguises itself as description:

> To my mind, therefore, it is a matter of great concern for all English users that several of our most eminent British linguists, grammarians in particular, have either overtly adopted prescription, or, by restricting the scope of what they describe and by using certain value-bearing terms as part of their description of English, are in part being covertly prescriptive. (p. 3)

Whereas the descriptive/prescriptive rub in linguistics is along nationalistic lines: American and British grammarians presenting a standardization of the language to themselves and to other speakers of English; the debate in anthropology is along world view distinctions with modernists and postmodernists debating the position of the observer as prescriptivist and as descriptivist (Clifford & Marcus, 1986; Crapanzano, 1986; Tyler, 1986). Tyler (1986, pp. 130–131) argues against description by pointing out the hierarchy implicit in the simple act of describing: The person who describes is in a position superior in some way to those who are described, or that which is described.

One way to avoid taking an authoritative position in research is to embrace what Lather (1986, p. 257) called "a democratized process of inquiry"—a process characterized by negotiation and reciprocity between the researcher and the researched. Another way is take part in what Keeney (1988, p. 102) characterizes as "Dostoyevskian dialogue," a process described as "a polyphony of many voices, none having the final word. Each voice has an opportunity to be heard, textualised, contextualised and decontextualised, as the listener desires. . . . A Dostoyevskian context allows any voice, but no final authoritarian voice" (p. 102).

Following this line of thought, a reader of the succeeding sections may interpret the words as an authoritarian, dictatorial voice on the standards of making a referral, or as only one voice in an ongoing dialogue or chorus on referrals, or as something all together different than what has been described above. The only authoritarian statement this author will make is that the spirit of the text follows the ethical imperative voiced by Heinz von Foerster (1984a, p. 60): "Act always so as to increase the number of choices." These words are offered as a choice, a difference, a path that may be followed, but the decision to follow cannot be located within these pages "because its meaning is not in it, but in an understanding, of which it is only a consumed fragment, it is no longer cursed with the task of representation" (Tyler, 1986, p. 129).

PRESCRIPTIONS FOR REFERRALS

Two recommendations previously made to physicians to improve communication in doctor-patient interaction have focused on the exchange of information between the two parties (Helman, 1985; Mathews, 1983; Stone, 1979; Waitzkin, 1985), and the role time plays in that exchange (Barnlund, 1984; Bruhn, 1986; Kreps & Thornton, 1984; Morrell, Evans, Morris, & Roland, 1986; Pluckham, 1978; Roland, Bartholomew, Courtenay, Morris, & Morrell, 1986). On the information side, researchers such as Waitzkin (1985) stated that doctors "tend to misperceive their own informative behavior and their patient's desire for information" (p. 99). Mathews (1983) added that this misperception was attributable to what she called "the incongruent frames of reference about what information ought to be shared" (p. 1371).

Evans et al. (1986) went further to highlight the need for awareness of frames of reference:

> The fundamental starting point of any diagnosis and treatment is comprehension—of the patient by the physician, and of the physician of the patient. The physician has a teaching function as well as a healing function to perform. But to be an effective teacher, the physician must discover not only the root causes of the patient's medical problem but also something of the conceptual structure that supports both the patient's and the doctor's perceptions and understanding of the problem and the task at hand. These must be managed as surely as any organic manifestation of disorder. Physicians must understand what is fundamental in the patient's comprehension of the problem. (p. 1033)

Dym (1987) continued the discussion of doctor-patient communication by stressing a more dynamic view of the information/frame process. Working form a cybernetic perspective, Dym stressed the recursive relationship inherent in information exchange. Whereas Evans and his colleagues (Evans et al., 1986) tended to highlight a static view of frames, Dym pushed for an understanding based on "the ongoing relationship between a continually adjusting system and its changing environment" (p. 37).

The simple request to exchange more information, with the hope that this increase will necessarily reduce uncertainty on the part of the patient and the physician, misses the point: In a recursive relationship, bits of information inform, and are informed by a context. Failure to grasp this pattern will usually mean that the participants will increase the amount of information in hopes of bringing about change, but this change results in a *more of the same* scenario. Dym's paper, grounded in the work of Bateson (1972) and Keeney (1983), and Evans and his colleagues emphasis on frames (Goffman, 1974), provide a firm foundation for the use of Recursive Frame Analysis (RFA) not only to describe the patterns of exchanging information, but also to prescribe ways in which the patterns can be altered.

The *more of the same* mentality is also a trap into which some of the proponents of increasing time spent between doctors and patients fall. An increase in the amount of time spent between doctors and patients without a focus on change in communication patterns is doomed to failure. Kreps and Thornton (1984) and others (Barnlund, 1984; Bruhn, 1986) stressed the importance of understanding the relationship between time and communication, the formal study of which is called chronemics. Kreps and Thornton (1984) stated that "time is, perhaps, the form of nonverbal communication that people are the least aware of, yet time has a major impact on human interaction" (p. 37). The point being that patterns of time and communication, or patterns of communication over time, are different than measuring the quantity of time spent communicating. Changes in the ways people interact may result in an increase in the amount of time the two parties spend together, or changes in the amount of time spent together may change the ways in which people interact, but the emphasis is on change in patterns, not on changes in the quantity of time.

In Chapter 4, RFA was employed as a way to describe the organization of patterns of communication as presented by the families during their interviews. Patterns of communication, discussed as frames and galleries, were created through the use of RFA to draw distinctions in the discourse. The emphasis was on presenting a picture or record of how the interviews could be understood. RFA can be used to manage and organize talk in real time: During face-to-face interaction, distinctions are drawn by speakers and listeners and these acts shape and are shaped by the ongoing flow of discourse (Keeney, 1990a, 1990b).

In the next section, a variety of RFA distinctions will be presented to suggest ways in which physicians and patients can "construct, deconstruct, relate, and manage frames" (Keeney, 1990b) during the referral process. From the study, one family's experiences will be used to illustrate how RFA distinctions can be used to help physicians and families manage communication during the referral process.

RFA PRESCRIPTIONS

In RFA, the basic notions are (a) frames, (b) gallery, (c) openings, and (d) embedding (Keeney, 1990b). In therapy, these distinctions are used "for both post hoc analyses of whole sessions and as a tool for organizing real-time therapeutic participation in an ongoing case" (Keeney, 1990a, p. 41). The first of the two functions (post hoc analysis) was used in Chapter 4 to create basic distinctions in the talk of the families about their experiences during the referral process. The second of these two functions (organizing real-time participation) will be used in this chapter to show ways in which participants in the referral process can organize and manage the information in which they are emersed.

Eliciting Frames

Frame elicitation is one the basic notions of RFA. It is an act or request for information. The information, in the form of discourse, is a building block for all of the other processes in RFA. In a therapy session, the clinician begins by eliciting information from the clients. The resulting frames or surface evidence (Tannen, 1979) help the therapist understand how the clients are organizing/constructing their world. The process would seem to be the same for the physician when interviewing a patient.

> We may not be able to know precisely what the patient's actual understanding of physiology or symptomology might be, but we often see in the patient's verbalization of conclusions or interferences that a characteristic kind of reasoning is at work. (Evans et al., 1986, p. 1031)

Each patient, physician, and family member has a particular way of expressing their world view (Becker, 1984b, 1988). One purpose of conversation is to try to understand each individual's use of language, and another intent is to try to understand what those utterances mean to the speaker and to the listeners. It is a complicated endeavor to accomplish, but a much needed one in such an important conversation as that which takes place between the doctor and the patient.

The purpose of frame elicitation is to allow the participants to investigate differences between their constructions. Agar (1985, p. 133) terms this process as discovering differences between institutional frames and client frames. The doctor, by virtue of being a member of the medical profession, has a different context than a parent, who has membership in another context, their family. The shape of a person's talk is the result of many contexts or restraints, and a professional membership can be an important one (Becker, 1984a, 1984b, 1988).

The doctor can elicit frames from the patient in order to hear how the patient is organizing the information at hand. This information can consist of many forms: How the family members understand the child's illness; how the family members comprehend the doctor's directions; or how the family members perceive the child now that the physician has introduced the frames of *heart murmur* and *referral to pediatric cardiologist* into the presenting gallery of *healthy child*. Given the ongoing recursion inherent in the information/frame cycle of communication, the elicitation of frames is necessitated throughout the entire referral process.

It is also important for the participants to remember that act of eliciting may help to change that which is being elicited. The form of the question is another context shaping the answer received (Becker, 1984a, 1884b, 1988). The unique questions asked by each family is a challenge to the physician, as commonly know information about heart murmurs is reshaped in order to answer the new request of the family. The same holds for the family members. The types of questions asked by the physician call for reshaping of what might have been familiar information to the family member. Because the request for information might be in an unfamiliar form, the old information needs to be reworked so as to achieve some sort of fit with the new question. At any time during the process, the patterns constructing the gallery of healthy child can be altered such that the context for understanding the child is changed, possibly to a gallery of *unhealthy child*. The simple asking of a question can accomplish that shift.

One routine doctors can adopt is that nothing is routine when communicating medical information to people who are not medically trained. A physician's framing of a referral to a pediatric cardiologist as routine might be questionable from a parent's perspective. The process by which a doctor's gallery for what is routine was built would be much different from a parent's construction of that gallery. The only way to bridge the difference is through the elicitation of frames.

If the family's understandings or frames are ignored problems can arise when the physician attempts to contextualize events in a way that is radically different from how the family perceives those events. "When the text [i.e., the diagnosis or referral] fails to match the receiver's [the parents'] frames, an operation of frame defense may ensue: The text is rejected or simply not understood in order to preserve the validity of the frames" (Beaugrande, 1980, p. 168). Hein and Wodak (1987) call this process "frame conflict" (p. 39) and Wadsworth (1976) believes that when this lack of understanding exists, patients are simply unable to listen to what physicians have to say to them. The same could be said for doctors too. Frame elicitation is one way to find out when there is a great difference between the patient's and the physician's understanding of a diagnosis or procedure.

Evans and his colleagues (Evans et al., 1986) discussed three instances when miscommunication could occur: (a) when there was an "absence of shared frames" (p. 1029); (b) when there was confusion or misframing on the part of the physician or patient (p. 1030); or (c) when there was a problem finding "a label to associate with the symptoms, perhaps to fill in a frame, or to find an organizing principle around which to structure a frame" (p. 1031).

In Chapter 4, there were many examples of these types of differences in content to frame or frame to frame relations (Keeney, 1990b). Individuals, whether medically trained or not, would have unique differences in how information is organized for the same concept (e.g., heart and referral). These differences were shaped by the individuals' prior experiences: interaction with medical personnel, personal health history, and television or print media sources. Depending on the parents' exposure to matters of the heart or medical encounters in general, there might have been some major differences between the family members' constructions and those of the referring physicians:

Parents' Heart Gallery	
F: Healthy	F: Unhealthy
f: no abnormalities	f: heart disease
	f: heart murmur

Physicians' Heart Gallery	
F: Healthy Heart	F: Unhealthy Heart
f: normal abnormalities	f: heart disease
f: innocent heart murmur	f: organic or pathological heart murmur

Both of these constructions could have also contrasted with a pediatric cardiologist's construction of the heart, especially with regard to murmurs (McNamara, 1987a, pp. 3–5):

Pediatric Cardiologist
F: Healthy Heart (with innocent heart murmur)
f: Neonatal pulmonary artery murmur
f: Still's Murmur
f: Pulmonary Valve Flow Murmur
f: Venous Hum

Parents may have thought of the heart only in terms of normal/healthy heart or abnormal/unhealthy heart. A heart murmur was an abnormality, therefore, their child had an unhealthy heart. This parent's construction would contrast with a physician's framing which would contextualize a murmur, not associated with any disease or abnormality of the heart, as a "normal variant" (McNamara, 1987a, p. 3). The only way a physician would be able to discern if the parent was framing an innocent heart murmur as abnormal/unhealthy, rather than normal variant/healthy, would be to elicit frames from the parents in order to hear their discriminations. The physician would have to pay close attention to any talk of the parents which would suggest a shift to an unhealthy/vulnerable child gallery: Examples of which would suggest an abnormal/unhealthy framing of the innocent heart murmur. When such frames were uttered, physicians would then have to react with frames of their own to help the family member recontextualize the murmur to shift the talk back to a healthy child gallery.

It is quite a challenge to track the sequence of frames in a session. Frames being elicited are only understood in the context of previously elicited frames. In RFA terms, the notion of frames being perceived within other frames is called embeddedness (Keeney, 1990a, 1990b). The next section examines two embedding distinctions: chunking and weaving.

Weaving

Keeney (1990b, p. 29) states that "the purpose of therapy is to move discourse into a 'therapeutic gallery' where clients and therapist may experience and utilize their frames as a resource." The beginning talk of a therapy session is considered to be organized around a problem. The initial gallery is called a problem gallery. By eliciting frames, embedding, and shifting the talk, the therapist attempts to change patterns in the talk until the discourse moves into what can be considered a therapeutic gallery.

The shifts in talk can be accomplished by what is called reframing (see Coyne, 1985). Reframing is said to occur when old information is understood within a new frame or context. Coyne (1985) stated that reframing involved "shifting the perspective within which a client experiences a situation in a way that fits the 'facts' of the situation as well, but that changes its entire meaning" (p. 337). For example, with systemic therapy, a sequence of events described by family members as problematic (old frame) comes to be described as being resourceful (new frame) for the family. As old frames are reframed, and as new frames are elicited, the talk shifts from the presenting or problematic gallery to a therapeutic gallery.

Once the discourse shifts to the so-called therapeutic gallery, the therapist strives to keep the talk within the context which has been constructed through the course of therapy. As new information is brought forth, the therapist must help the client weave the new threads of discourse into the existing tapestry: the therapeutic gallery. Keeney (1990a, p. 77) states that weaving in therapy "invokes taking whatever frame the client proposes and utilizing it as further evidence that their conversation belongs within a particular gallery." The new frames become embedded into old frames that have been arranged into a therapeutic gallery.

With the referring physicians and the family members, sometimes the reverse process occurred: discourse shifted from a nonproblematic gallery (healthy child), to a problematic one (unhealthy child). A family brought their child in for routine checkups and their perspective or presenting gallery was that of a healthy child. But when frames such as heart murmur and referral to a heart specialist were introduced, some families had trouble fitting those frames into the gallery of healthy child. The result of these shifts was that some families shifted their perspective to a gallery (unhealthy child) in which they could fit the frames of murmur/referral.

With some families, those frames created openings or leaks (Keeney,

1990b) in the families' presenting galleries. An opening would be a frame which opens a door out of a particular gallery. With the heart murmur, if the parents perceived that their child's heart murmur was of a serious nature, that would be an opening into a new gallery, possibly a problematic one. When that happened, physicians had to work very hard to shift the talk back into a therapeutic or nonproblematic gallery.

The next two examples (Excerpts XX and YY) demonstrate the efforts of one physician and her colleagues had to undertake in order to help the parents shift their talk back into the healthy child gallery. In XX, the interviewer asked the father why he was not very worried about the referral to the cardiologist (Lines 01-03). The father confirmed that talking with the referring physician's colleagues had been helpful (Line 04), and the mother also acknowledged the role the physician's colleagues had in helping the family (Lines 05–07) by describing the efforts the doctors made "they came in there and stayed about 10 minutes or so just talking to us."

Excerpt XX

(01) *I:* Craig, I know you said you weren't that worried, you feel pretty
(02) optimistic about it. Was it helpful for you though too having the
(03) practitioners there and hearing what they had to say?
(04) *F:* Yeah.
(05) *M:* Cause they they're more vocal than the doctor. I guess they must
(06) have more time than the doctor, cause after she left and they
(07) came in stayed in there about 10 minutes or so just talking to us.

Later in the discussion (Excerpt YY), the mother went on to give more details about the conversations the doctors had with the parents after the referring physician left. From the mother's description, it was clear that the associates were attempting to weave the new frames of heart murmur and referral such that the frames would fit within the parents presenting gallery of healthy child.

Excerpt YY

(01) *M:* I was really scared. I don't think Craig was very afraid, but I was
(02) really scared that something was real, real serious. But she [the
(03) referring physician] talked well besides the doctor talking to us
(04) she has two neo-natal practitioners and specialists. And all three
(05) of them came in and talked with us. And all three of them kept
(06) assuring us that it was nothing major, but they didn't know what
(07) it was.
(08) *I:* Did that reduce the anxiety or increase it because there were
(09) three of them
(10) *M:* No it reduced it, it helped.
(11) *I:* Okay. So that did help.
(12) *M:* Yeah especially by the time the third one talked to us. That really
(13) helped.

In Lines 05 through 07, the mother stated, "all three of them [the referring physician's associates] kept assuring us that it was nothing major, but they didn't know what it was." The first move in that quote was a reframing attempt on the part of the associates. The frames of heart murmur and referral were being embedded within a larger frame of *nothing major:*

F: Nothing major
  f: heart murmur
f: referral.

From the excerpt, it seemed that the associates were attempting to weave the frames such that there would be a better fit with the healthy child gallery, and also, any leaks or openings to the unhealthy child gallery would be patched up.

As the mother recalled, it took about 10 minutes and three associates (two neonatal practitioners and another specialist) to patch up the leak. In taking a closer look at what the doctors were saying, it was quite clear why it took so long to weave the problematic frames into a healthy child gallery: Each time the doctors reframed the murmur/referral frame as being "nothing major," they then presented another opening for the parents to take: "but they [the doctors] didn't know what it [the child's heart murmur] was" (Lines 06 and 07). By using a *Yes . . . , but* sequence, the doctors were creating a side-by-side pattern:

F: Nothing major / F: But they don't know what it is
  (Weaving in   (Opening to G: Unhealthy child)
G: Healthy child),

or worse yet, the *didn't know* frame could have been interpreted as a reframing of nothing major:

G: Healthy child
  F: But we don't know what it is / F: Nothing major
    f: heart murmur
    f: referral
G: Unhealthy child.

If the doctors had reworded their reframings to a *Yes . . . , and* pattern, then their task of weaving/patching might have been less time-consuming. A *yes . . . ,* and reframe would have allowed the parents to contextualize the *we don't know what it is* as falling under the *nothing major* frame:

F: Nothing major
  f: They didn't know what it was and it's nothing major.

Some observers might argue that such a minor move like the one presented above would not be enough to shift families out of one gallery and into another, or to help families maintain their current gallery. It is important to remember that even subtle shifts in meaning can be very influential, especially, if the listener is in a situation that is being perceived as extremely important, even life-threatening. A consult, with a doctor over their child's heart, demands close listening on the part of the parents, as well as careful speaking on the part of the physician. The close scrutiny on the part of the parents is a resource for the referring physician. With careful wording, the doctor can effectively persuade the family members not to worry. Of course, the physician must also recognize times when parents are too distraught to hear what is being said. At those times, it would behoove the physician to elicit frames from the parents in order to evaluate what had and what had not been understood by the parents. It may require allowing some time to pass in order for the family members to work through the information, before the physician can better know how the members have contextualized the new frames.

The doctor and her associates, discussed in Excerpts XX and YY, seemed to give the parents some extra time after hearing the news of the murmur and the referral. The doctor, in her practice, appeared to be quite willing to give families opportunities to contact her in order to discuss concerns that would arise during the referral process.

Excerpt ZZ

(01) *M:* Right, cause I've told other people that that's one of the reasons
(02) that I really like Dr. Carlisle cause she has. You know the stuff
(03) where you'd be afraid to call the doctor and think "this isn't a
(04) thing to call the doctor." And you can call those two on their
(05) beepers and they'll call you back in 10 minutes every time. So
(06) they're a, I think they're a real plus.

In the preceding example (ZZ), the mother stated that the doctor was always available to talk with her about the family's concerns. The doctor appeared to have created a context in which it made sense for parents to ask questions about treatment (Lines 01–04). This doctor provided the parents with the opportunity to present their concerns. Or, in other words, the doctor encouraged the parents to present their frames. With these frames, the doctor would be able to hear how families were doing and also, it would allow the doctor to react if the therapeutic gallery had leaked.

Maintaining Galleries

Galleries can leak at any time. Even though the families leave the doctor's office firmly entrenched in a therapeutic gallery, the environment of the family provides ample opportunities for new frames to be introduced. These new frames may result in leaks happening in the galleries.

As was seen in Chapter 4, families experienced leaks and openings: by consulting medical reference books (Excerpt EE); by reading pamphlets in the specialist's office (Excerpt FF); by talking with friends and relatives (Excerpts GG and HH); and by the referring physicians themselves (Excerpts D, E, and F). Doctors and therapists alike need to be aware when galleries begin to leak: Utterances and behaviors of the physician or therapist can be understood differently, depending on the perspective(s)/galleries of the family members. If a leak has occurred, family members' understandings of the process of referral and diagnosis can be radically altered.

One way for physicians to help maintain therapeutic galleries is to encourage interaction with their patients. The doctor, described in Excerpts YY–ZZ, seemed to provide many occasions during the referral process when the parents could have contacted her. These contacts would have provided the doctor with opportunities to elicit frames and to weave these frames such that a therapeutic gallery could be maintained.

In Excerpt AAA, this process was used to help the mother and her family maintain the healthy child gallery. With the visit to the heart specialist coming up soon, the mother was as concerned for her child's health, and was keeping close scrutiny over her child's activities and well-being. A *rash* was discovered on the child and the mother's mother suggested that it might be a *staph infection*. The framing of a rash as a staph infection was a sign that there were times that the family was operating from an unhealthy child gallery:

G: Healthy child / G: Unhealthy child
  F: rash / F: staph infection.

The mother called the doctor and reported her concern. The doctor seemed to be able to weave the rash/staph infection frame such that the healthy child gallery was maintained and the opening to the unhealthy child gallery was closed off for the time being:

G: Healthy child
  F: "I don't think you really have anything to worry about. Everything will be fine."
    f: rash.

The mother, upon hearing this weaving, was able to repeat the message to her daughter, and between the mother and the doctor, the daughter was also able to stay within the healthy child gallery: "when I got off the phone, Amy [the daughter] was going, "She [the doctor] says everything's okay." Another leak was patched.

Excerpt AAA

M: No. Cause my mother's really and my daughter the only one's
really knew. I they thought (( )). My daughter was
understandably upset, because she didn't understand either, being
13. But you know what really helped her was that I called uh . . I
kinda of overacted and I thought he had maybe a rash. And my
mother said, "No it's a staph infection." "So we called the
practitioner". And I'm telling her "Well I'm kind of overreacting
cause I'm kind of worried about Monday."
I: Um Hum.
M: And then she said again, "Well, you know I don't think you
really have anything to worry about. Everything will be fine."
And when my daughter, I must have repeated her, cause when I
got off the phone, Amy was going, "She says everything's okay."
And then she was fine after that. After she had heard me
repeating it, even though (she heard it in) the doctor's office.

WAYS OF WEAVING AND MAINTAINING

There are a variety of approaches through which physicians can assist patients in the process of weaving in new frames and maintaining therapeutic galleries. Physicians can discuss matters through face-to-face interaction or by the use of telephone conversations. Examples of these two methods were illustrated in this chapter (see Excerpts XX, YY, ZZ, AAA).

In addition, physicians can utilize written hand-outs for families to take home and to read when concerns arise. Dr. Daniel McNamara (1987a) developed a concise pamphlet for families with children who have had diagnosed innocent heart murmurs. In the hand-out, McNamara acknowledged and normalized the worry family members went through during the discovery of an innocent heart murmur. He also confirmed the confusing nature of murmurs and then he went through a series of steps to help parents and patients discriminate between innocent and pathological murmurs (p. 2).

F: Innocent murmur (functional or benign mumurs)	F: Organic murmur (Pathological murmur)
f: not associated with any disease	f: due to either birth defect or
f: not associated with any abnormality of the heart	f: acquired disease of the heart

McNamara concluded his written explanation by underlining the importance of maintaining a healthy child gallery:

> Once your doctor determines that a heart murmur is innocent and that an extra sound is normal, it is no longer necessary to check it nor should the child be restricted or be given any special precautions. Substituting the word "normal" for "innocent" may be the best way to think about it. That alone should guide management of the child who has one of these sounds which, if not appropriately ignored, can plague a child's life. (p. 7)

Besides these methods, physicians can also use consultants such as counselors, therapists, or other health care practitioners on the staff as those who can either sit down with the families or be available for telephone calls in order to discuss family members' questions or concerns. The physician in this study (Excerpt CC) used her associates to help weave the families' frames so as to patch opening openings arising from the referral to the pediatric cardiologist. Also, the parents recalled how the referring physicians' colleagues helped to lend support to the family during their time of worry and concern.

All of these approaches suggested in this chapter as ways to help doctors help family members through the ordeal of referral evoke an image of heart murmurs, which is often overlooked: the interactional nature of disease.

INTERACTIONAL NATURE OF HEART MURMURS

Engel (1977) and Dym (1987) are just two of many authors (e.g., Andersen & Naess, 1986; Dracup & Melies, 1982; Stone, 1979; Szasz & Hollender, 1956) who have advocated an interactional view of medicine. The notion of interaction advocated by Engel and Dym involved a systems view of the embedded nature of biological, social, and psychological frames.

> The dominant model of disease today is biomedical, and it leaves no room within its framework for the social, psychological, and behavioral dimensions of illness. A biopsychosocial model is proposed that provides a blueprint for research, a framework for teaching, and a design for action in the real world of health care. (Engel, 1977, p. 135)

Dym expanded Engel's approach by discussing how taking an interactional view allows for different perspectives to be considered when conceptualizing the recursive relationship between the context and that which is contextualized:

> The ways that professionals manage an illness and that families cope with and adapt to an illness can all be shown to influence the shape and duration of its biological course. The onset, course, and treatment of illness also have a powerful impact on individual patients, other family members, and family systems. (Dym, 1987, p. 35)

Others (e.g., Andersen & Naess, 1986; Szasz & Hollender, 1956), also followed this line of thinking by stating that interaction does not necessarily mean relationships between disciplines or recognized world views, but rather relationships between people. Andersen and Naess (1986) "find it useful to think of the heart in relational terms: The heart is part of a person who is part of relationships." For the patients in this study, they were not only in relationships with mother, father, sister and brothers, but also with doctors—physicians who had to interact with the child and the child's heart to diagnose the nature of the heart murmur.

> The concept of a relationship is a novel one in medicine. Traditionally, physicians have been concerned with "things," for example, anatomical structures, lesions, bacteria, and the like. In modern times the scope has been broadened to include the concept of "function." The phenomenon of a human relationship is often viewed as though it were a "thing" or a "function." It is in fact, neither. Rather it is an abstraction, appropriate for the description, and handling of certain observational facts. Moreover, it is an abstraction which presupposes concepts of both structure and function. (Szasz & Hollender, 1956, pp. 385–386)

When it is time to identify an abstraction as an "innocent heart murmur," the doctor is concerned with the structure and function of the heart, but the meaning of the murmur as abstraction is embodied in the relationship between the child, the doctor, and the parents. The child's heart sits close to the front wall of the chest. The chest wall is thin and sounds are more easily heard by a listener (McNamara, 1987a, p. 3). During examinations, children fidget and squirm; they cry and fuss. There are noises in the room. All these interfere with the doctor's painstaking care to hear and identify the murmur.

The amount of practice that a physician has in identifying murmurs is also figured into the heart murmur as abstraction. "In a short office visit, some murmurs take time to figure out even for the most skilled and experienced of physicians and might require another examination or special tests and sometimes consultation with a pediatric cardiologist" (McNamara, 1987a, p. 3). The identification can involve listening to the heart, reading test results, and consulting with other medical personnel.

Intertwined with all of this is the use of language: Diagnoses, procedures, and concerns all exist in language, too. The frames of the physicians and the family members interact to produce meaning for the heart murmur abstraction.

> When we consider a relationship in which there is joint participation of the two persons involved, "relationship" refers to neither a structure nor a function (such as the "personality" of the physician or patient). It is, rather, an abstraction embodying the activities of two interacting systems (persons). (Szasz & Hollender, 1956, p. 586)

A murmur may be only a sound, but that sound in the heart takes on meaning in the minds, and in the language, of parents, patients, and physicians. In such a process, listening to participants' frames is a crucial as hearing hearts' sounds.

FUTURE STUDIES

As a research study, this text accomplished two major goals: (a) to address major concerns in the area of families' understandings of heart murmur referrals; and (b) to raise new questions about families, referrals, and the practice of medicine. The latter of these two goals, the raising of new questions, is the focus of this section. This discussion will not only address issues of what next to study in this area, but also how to study these concerns.

A next, logical step in the study of referrals to cardiologists would be to compare and contrast families' interpretations based upon differences in initial diagnoses of the identified patient (Chenail, 1988; Park et al., 1988). Families could be grouped by diagnosis to see how the severity of the heart condition would shape the discourse of the family. For example, how would patterns of discovery, diagnosis, and referral differ for families with children who have been diagnosed as having heart defects more serious (e.g., cyanotic heart disease, non-cyanotic heart disease with a history of congestive heart failure, etc.) (Park et al., 1988) as compared to families with children who have been diagnosed as having heart murmurs?

Another related study would be to examine families' reactions to other types of referrals: How do families interpret referrals to other specialists (e.g., Amir, 1987; Gidding & Rosenthal, 1984), to mental health counselors (e.g., Good, Good, & Cleary, 1987; Mackenzie, 1982; Schwenk, 1987; Yaffe & Stewart, 1986), to family therapists, or to other doctors, so as to seek second opinions (e.g., Brenner et al., 1984)?

Directionality of these referrals could be studied: Are there differences in interpretations when a family therapist refers a family to a physician as compared to when a medical doctor suggests family therapy for patients?

Besides scrutinizing families and their interpretations during the referral process, investigators can also conduct interviews with families after they have met with the cardiologists/specialists (Chenail, 1988; Park et al., 1988). Such an investigation could focus on the resiliency of families' frames: Do parents hold on to vulnerable child frames even after a pediatric cardiologist has cleared the organic murmur frames, or are parents able to shift their talk out of a problem gallery and into a therapeutic gallery?

In addition to studying families' talk about the talk in referral consults with physicians, researchers could also gain access to tapes and transcripts of the talk which occurred while the physician was actually making the referral. The same could be done with the consults made with the specialists (Chenail, 1988). The organization of these talks could be examined; comparisons could be made between families' interpretations and the transcripts of the actual sessions; and/or doctors' theories about referrals/consults could be compared to the doctors' talk in the sessions in order to learn more about how doctors put theory into practice.

Researchers could also choose to apply different methodologies to the study of referrals. Whereas this project incorporated one type of discourse analysis (recursive frame analysis), other researchers can chose another variety of discourse analysis (see Tracy, 1988), or any of number of qualitative methods (see Keeney & Morris, 1985a, 1985b). In addition, quantitative and qualitative approaches can be combined so as to produce what Jick (1983) referred to as "triangulation in action" (p. 135).

In contrast to the discovery-oriented approach taken in this study (see Mahrer, 1988), researchers can take a hypothesis-testing perspective (i.e., Keppel, 1982; Kerlinger, 1986) to confirm or disconfirm theoretical positions on the topic of referrals. Hypothesis-testing research can also be combined with descriptive/discovery-oriented research to produce interesting results (see Hopper, 1988). The only limits to how a topic can be studied are the restrictions, either knowingly or unknowingly, placed there by the researchers themselves.

One matter left unresolved at this point is how an investigator should disseminate the ideas and conclusions of this or any project (see Backer, Liberman, & Kuehnel, 1986). Usual procedures dictate that the academician write and present the findings of studies to other academicians so as to aid in the progress of knowledge (Kerlinger, 1986). Other researchers who have studied medical communication have been criticized for writing and publishing only for their peers (other researchers), rather than presenting the findings to physicians and other medical personnel (Rogers, 1987, p. 694). Another concerned party, who is usually excluded from the information dissemination, are the parents, patients, and other family members who have, and will have, additional experiences with physicians and the medical systems. The question here is should researchers be the only ones privy to the findings of their research, or should the researched also have access to the results and findings.

Sometimes writing for popular journals and even magazines can be hazardous for the academician's career (i.e., when being evaluated for tenure or promotions). The argument here is for responsible research which entails attempts by researchers to reach those nonacademic persons who indeed have vested interests in these observations. One way to address this concern is to create dialogue with the subjects of a study; make findings available for the families who were studied, while at the same time, protecting the confidentiality of the subjects. This process for this project is being carried out through another phase of the research: Families from the study are being contacted to hear of the results of their consults with the pediatric cardiologists, and also to provide an opportunity to ask parents if they would be interested in receiving a written summary of the findings of the first phase of the project, the interviews discussed in this text.

Another way to disseminate these findings to a wider audience is by preparing an article to be submitted to a popular, family-oriented journal such as *Good Housekeeping*. It is important to remember that magazines like *Good Housekeeping* are not only an important source of medical information for families, but the publishers of these magazines also publish medical guides for families [e.g., *Good Housekeeping Family Health & Medical Guide* (1979); *Better Homes and Gardens New Family Medical Guide* (Kiester, Jr., 1982), etc.]. As was seen in this study (see Excerpt EE), families do consult these reference books for information on medical issues, such as the discovery of a heart murmur. It is important to become involved in these sources of information because they are used by many people in the creation of contexts, contexts in which they live their lives.

IMPLICATIONS OF THE STUDY

When discussing the implications of this or any research project, the question arises, "What was the worth or value of the study?" After all the distinctions have been drawn, after all the analyses have been stated, what then about the project can the investigator claim to be significant? The issue of significance, in this case, is not a statistical one, but rather, a matter of difference.

By difference, I am referring to the Batesonian conceptualization of the term. The following excerpt should shed light on how the notion of difference is related to significance. When discussing Kant's position, that even in a simple piece of chalk there are a multitude of potential facts, Bateson (1972) wrote

> There is an infinite number of *differences* [emphasis from original] around and within the piece of chalk. There are differences between the chalk and the rest of the universe, between the chalk and the sun or the moon. And within the piece of chalk, there is for every molecule an infinite number of differences between its location and the locations in which it *might* [emphasis from original] have been. Of this infinitude, we select a very limited number, which become information In fact, what we mean by information—the elementary unit of information—is a *difference which makes a difference* [emphasis from original]. (p. 453)

The significance of a study, therefore, is understood in terms of the relationship between information and difference: The findings of a study, which made a difference in how we came to know the subject matter, would be considered information, as well as being significant. The challenge posed at the beginning of this report was, "By studying parents' discourse from a systemic family therapy perspective, what can we learn about parents' understandings of their child's heart murmur?" Now that the project has been completed, the question remains: What do we know differently about heart murmurs, health communication/discourse studies, and systemic family therapy?

Heart Murmurs

A crucial point of this study was that, although the diagnosis of a child's innocent heart murmur may be readily understood by a physician, the meaning of the murmur's discovery may be unclear to the parents. The nature of the heart murmur may be further obscured when the child is subsequently referred to a pediatric cardiologist. There is ambiguity inherent in the notion of referable innocent heart murmur. On one hand, a referable heart murmur is insignificant because the act of referral is only a formality: The referring physician only wishes to confirm the innocence of the murmur. But, on the other hand, murmurs are referable because there may be a question of heart defects and heart disease, and only a heart specialist could answer those concerns. So with the referable heart murmur, the parents have to make a choice: Is the murmur serious or not?

The choice may not be a simple one. If the referring physician knows enough about the heart murmur to identify the sound as a sign of innocence, then why must the child be referred? What prevents the doctor from making a definitive diagnosis? The doctor may say that a referral is routine, but if the physician does not know enough about the heart to make a diagnosis, does the doctor know enough to know what he or she does not know? Maybe the doctor could not know if there was something seriously wrong with the child's heart, or maybe the doctor is withholding something from the parents?

Part of the confusion, and possibly the worry, surrounding the nature of a referable heart murmur results from the parents' questioning of the expertise of the physician: Can physicians be experts on what they do and do not know? The framing of the referral is crucial. In some way, the referral should be contextualized as a normal course of action, and an indication of how the physician is acting as an expert.

If the doctor can help the parents maintain a context in which the referral is understood as being routine, then there will probably be a good chance that the parents will not begin to view and/or treat their child as being vulnerable or suffering from heart disease. If the nature of the referral is unclear to the parents or they understand the referral as being an indication that something is seriously wrong with the child, then the parents may begin to contextualize their child as being unhealthy.

Given all the possible interpretations that may arise from a referral for an innocent heart murmur, it would behoove the pediatric cardiologist to investigate the parents' understanding of their child's condition when the families arrive at the clinic. Besides diagnosing the heart murmur, the specialist may also have to treat the context in which the heart murmur was understood by the parents. Part of this treatment would involve demonstrating to the parents that there is not an *either/or* relationship between innocent heart murmurs and healthy children (e.g., A child is either healthy, or the child has a heart murmur.), but rather, that a *both/and* relationship exists between innocent heart murmurs and children's overall health (e.g., A child can be both healthy, and have an innocent heart murmur too.).

Health Communication and Discourse Analysis

This research continues the growing trend of utilizing discourse analysis in examining health communication. At the same time, the study also makes an original contribution to the field: By selecting an area of concern which had not been previously studied from a communication/discourse perspective (e.g., parents' talk about their child's heart murmur); by demonstrating the usefulness of an interview format in studying parents' narratives (e.g., creating a context for variation and diversity in parents' stories); and by studying conversational organization with Recursive Frame Analysis.

Prior to this research project, there had been only one detailed study of parental reaction to children's heart murmurs (Bergman & Stamm, 1967), but this research represents the only attempt at making a close-textual study in order to draw finer distinctions about parents' understandings and reactions to having a child be referred to a pediatric cardiologist. The results of this endeavor point to the importance of assessing the subtle, and not so subtle signs—ways in which an innocent heart murmur can be understood.

Great effort was taken in conducting the parental interviews so as to create a balance between consistency and diversity across the parents' accounts of their experiences with the heart murmur discovery-referral process. The challenge of using an interview format is that there needs to be enough structure in the interaction between participants so as to allow for comparisons to be made across interviews, but the ordering of inquires can not be so rigid or leading that parents' particularities are severely restrained.

The use of Recursive Frame Analysis to study health communication was somewhat of a departure from previous utilizations of the method. Prior to this study, RFA had been used primarily to organize therapeutic discourse in systemic family therapy sessions. Especially significant in this application of RFA was the introduction of the notion of predetermined galleries as a way to conceptualize making comparisons across different interviews. The notion of predetermined galleries permitted necessary structure for the post-hoc analysis of the parents' narratives (e.g., All interviews would have mention of heart murmur discoveries.), and, at the same time, diversity of parents' stories could be studied from a common perspective.

As stated above, RFA had been primarily used in clinical practice, where its concise nature had been of great utility in providing brief pictures of the conversational organization of a session. Contributions made by this study include further development of RFA as a formalized research approach, establishment of RFA's place within a larger/older research tradition, description of RFA conventions in inquiry and presentation, and development of cross-case comparisons using RFA. Although there is much to be done before RFA is in a form that would allow for more rigorous studies in the mode of the Natural History of an Interview-type approach, it can be seen from this endeavor that the parsimonious way in which RFA permits basic distinctions to be made in discourse suggests that it would be beneficial to continue with the development of RFA as a research method.

Systemic Family Therapy

As mentioned above, RFA had been primarily used in making descriptions and prescriptions in systemic family therapy sessions. The utilization of RFA as a formalized research approach may provide future opportunities for investigations into therapeutic process. Besides contributing possible research applications to systemic family therapy, this project also helps to create new opportunities for the therapist in the medical area.

This study has shown the importance communication plays in the diagnosis and treatment of a condition such as an innocent heart murmur. Reading people's reactions to diagnoses can be as crucial to the successful outcome of treatment as is the interpretation of test results. How patients understand what is told to them in a doctor's office is a sometimes ignored in the normal course of medical treatment.

In contrast to this scenario is the emphasis systemic family therapists place on recognizing how clients contextualize what is being said during a therapy session. Describing patterns of process is the focus of this approach to therapy. The results of this study suggest that there may be substantial benefits in combining the communicational expertise of the systemic family therapist with the informational burdens of the medical doctor. Doctors may not have the time to sit down with family members and help them organize the information that has just been exchanged, but the inclusion of a systemic family therapist as a consultant in the process may help the families with the sometimes overwhelming amount of information and enable doctors to spend more time and effort on other medical matters.

CONCLUSION

When referring families with children who have suspected heart murmurs to pediatric cardiologists, physicians face a dilemma: They must build a context for referral so that going to see a heart specialist makes sense to a family, and at the same time, doctors must help a family maintain a context so that going to see a pediatric cardiologist does *not* mean that a child with an innocent heart murmur is unhealthy or vulnerable. Given the recursive process entailed in the construction of meaning, doctors are faced with a potentially neverending consult with patients in order to help maintain a gallery in which a referral is necessary, but is not cause for grave alarm on the part of family members.

This is not to say that parents do *not* have the right to worry about their child's health, nor that doctors have the ability to prevent this worry on the part of their patients or patients' families. No matter how the referral is presented, the importance of the heart almost necessitates a certain amount of worry (McNamara, personal communication, January 27, 1989). But the descriptions provided in the previous chapter do raise some important questions as to how referring physicians can prepare families for a referral such that the ordeal for a family is reduced.

References

Agar, M. (1979). Themes revisited: Some problems in cognitive anthropology. *Discourse Processes, 2*, 11–31.

Agar, M. (1985). Institutional discourse. *Text, 5*, 147–168.

The American Heritage Dictionary of the English Language (2nd ed.). (1970). New York: American Heritage Publishing.

Amir, M. (1987). Considerations guiding physicians when informing cancer patients. *Social Science & Medicine, 24*, 741–748.

Anderson, B. J., & Kornblum, H. (1984). The family environment of children with a diabetic parent: Issues for research. *Family Systems Medicine, 4*, 96–106.

Anderson, T., & Naess, I. (1986). Four hearts and four families in dilemma. *Family Systems Medicine, 4*, 96–106.

Ariel, S. (1987). An information processing theory of family dysfunction. *Psychotherapy, 24*, 477–495.

Aylward, G. P. (1988). Identification versus diagnosis: More than a semantic difference. *Journal of Pediatrics, 112*, 677.

Backer, T. E., Liberman, R. P., & Kuehnel, T. G. (1986). Dissemination and adoption of innovative psychosocial interventions. *Journal of Consulting and Clinical Psychology, 54*, 111–118.

Banta, H. D. (1983). Social science on medical technology: Utility and limitations. *Social Science & Medicine, 17*, 1363–1369.

Barnlund, D. C. (1984). The mystification of meaning: Doctor–patient encounters. In G. L. Kreps & B. C. Thornton (Eds.), *Health communication: Theory and practice* (pp. 39–50). New York: Longman. (Reprinted from *Journal of Medical Education*, 1976, *51*, 716–725)

Bateson, G. (1956). The message "This is play." In B. Schaffner (Ed.), *Group processes: Transactions of the second conference* (pp. 145–242). New York: Josiah Macy, Jr. Foundation.

Bateson, G. (1971). Chapter 1: Communication. In N. A. McQuown (Ed.), *The natural history of an interview* (pp. 1–40). (Available from Microfilm Collection of Manuscripts on Cultural Anthropology. Chicago: University of Chicago, Joseph Regenstein Library, Department of Photoduplication)

Bateson, G. (1972). *Steps to an ecology of mind*. New York: Ballantine Books.

Bateson, G. (1979). *Mind and nature: A necessary unity*. New York: Bantam Books.

Beaugrande, R. D. (1980). *Text, discourse, and process: Toward a multidisciplinary science of texts*. Norwood, NJ: Ablex.

Becker, A. L. (1984a). Biography of a sentence: A Burmese proverb. In S. Plattner (Ed.), *Text, play, and story: The construction and reconstruction of self and society* (1983 Proceedings of the American Ethnological Society) (pp. 135–155). Washington, DC: American Ethnological Society.

Becker, A. L. (1984b). The linguistics of particularity: Interpreting superordination in a Javanese text. In *Proceedings of the tenth annual meeting of the Berkeley Linguistics Society* (pp. 425–436). Berkeley, CA: Linguistics Department, University of California, Berkeley.

Becker, A. L. (1988). Language in particular: A lecture. In D. Tannen (Ed.), *Linguistics in context: Connecting observations and understanding: Lectures from the 1985 LSA/TESOL and NEH Institutes* (pp. 17–35). Norwood, NJ: Ablex.

Bergman, A. B., & Stamm, S. J. (1967). The morbidity of cardiac nondisease in school children. *New England Journal of Medicine, 276*, 1008–1013.

Bloch, D. A. (1986). The family therapist as consultant to health care organizations. In L. C. Wynne, S. H. McDaniel, & T. T. Weber (Eds.), *Systems consultation: A new perspective for family therapy* (pp. 139–149). New York: Guilford Press.

Brenner, J. I., Ringel, R. E., & Berman, M. A. (1984). Cardiological perspectives of chest pain in childhood: A referral problem? To whom? *Pediatric Clinics of North America, 31*, 1241–1258.

Bruhn, J. G. (1986). Time in therapeutic relationships: Myths and realities. *Southern Medical Journal, 79*, 344–350.

Buttny, R. (in press). Blame-accounts sequences in therapy: The negotiation of relational meanings. *Semiotica.*

Buttny, R., & Lannamann, J. W. (1986). *Framing problems: The hierarchial organization of discourse in a family therapy session.* Unpublished manuscript.

Caldwell, S. M., & Pichert, J. W. (1985). Systems theory applied to families with a diabetic child. *Family Systems Medicine, 3*, 34–44.

Cassata, D. M. (1978). Health communication theory and research: An overview of the communication specialist interface. In B. D. Ruben (Ed.), *Communication yearbook 2* (pp. 495–522). New Brunswick, NJ: Transaction Books.

Cassata, D. M. (1980). Health communication theory and research: A definitial overview. In D. Nimmo (Ed.), *Communication yearbook 4* (pp. 583–589). New Brunswick, NJ: Transaction Books.

Chenail, R. J. (1988). *Family system/medical system discourse: A recursive frame analysis.* Unpublished manuscript, Texas Tech University, Lubbock.

Clifford, J., & Marcus, G. E. (Eds.). (1986). *Writing culture: The poetics and politics of ethnography.* Berkeley, CA: University of California Press.

Coyne, J. C. (1985). Toward a theory of frames and reframing: The social nature of frames. *Journal of Marital and Family Therapy, 11*, 337–344.

Crapanzano, V. (1986). Hermes' dilemma: The masking of subversion in ethnographic description. In J. Clifford & G. E. Marcus (Eds.), *Writing cul-*

ture: *The poetics and politics of ethnography* (pp. 51–76). Berkeley, CA: University of California Press.
Davis, K. (1986). The process of problem (re)formulation in psychotherapy. *Sociology of Health & Illness, 8*, 44–74.
Di Pietro, R. J. (Ed.). (1982). *Linguistics and the professions: Proceedings of the second annual Delaware symposium on language studies*. Norwood, NJ: Ablex.
Doherty, W. J., & Baird, M. A. (1983). *Family therapy and family medicine: Toward the primary care of families*. New York: Guilford Press.
Doherty, W. J., & Baird, M. A. (Eds.). (1987). *Family-centered medical care*. New York: Guilford Press.
Dracup, K., & Meleis, A. I. (1982). Compliance: An interactionist approach. *Nursing Research, 31*, 31–36.
Dym, B. (1987). The cybernetics of physical illness. *Family Process, 26*, 35–48.
Engel, G. L. (1977). The need for a new medical model: A challenge for biomedicine. *Science, 196*, 129–136.
Evans, D. A., Block, M. R., Steinberg, E. R., & Penrose, A. M. (1986). Frames and heuristics in doctor-patient discourse. *Social Science & Medicine, 22*, 1027–1034.
Fairman, T. (1989). Let grammarians return to describing the language. *English Today, 5*, 3–5.
Feinstein, A. R., Taube, H., Cavalieri, R., Schultz, S. C., & Kryle, L. (1962). Physical activities and rheumatic heart disease in asymptomatic patients. *Journal of the American Medical Association, 180*, 1028–1031.
Fisher, S., & Todd, A. D. (Eds.). (1983). *The social organization of doctor-patient communication*. Washington, DC: Center for Applied Linguistics.
Fisher, S., & Todd, A. D. (Eds.). (1986). *Discourse and institutional authority: Medicine, education, and law*. Norwood, NJ: Ablex.
Fisher, W. R. (1987). *Human communication as narration: Toward a philosophy of reason, value, and action*. Columbia, SC: University of South Carolina Press.
Fisher, W. R. (1989). Clarifying the narrative paradigm. *Communication Monographs, 56*, 55–58.
Frankel, R. M. (1984a). From sentence to sequence: Understanding the medical encounter through microinteractional analysis. *Discourse Processes, 7*, 135–170.
Frankel, R. M. (Ed.). (1984b). Physicians and patients in social interaction: Medical encounters as a discourse process [Special issue]. *Discourse Processes, 7*.
Frawley, W. (1987a). Review article of *Handbook of discourse analysis*. *Language, 63*, 361–397.
Frawley, W. (1987b). *Text and epistemology*. Norwood, NJ: Ablex.
Freeman, S. H. (1987). Introduction. Verbal communication in medical encounters: An overview of recent work. *Text, 7*, 3–17.
Freeman, S. H., & Heller, M. S. (Eds.). (1987). Medical discourse [Special issue]. *Text, 7*.

Gephart, W. J. (1981). Watercolor painting. In N. L. Smith (Ed.), *Metaphors for evaluation: Sources of new methods* (pp. 247–272). Beverly Hills, CA: Sage.

Gidding, S. S., & Rosenthal, A. (1984). The interface between primary care and pediatric cardiology. *Pediatric Clinics of North America, 31*, 1367–1388.

Glaser, H. H., Harrison, G. S., & Lynn, D. B. (1964). Emotional implications of congenital heart disease in children. *Pediatrics, 34*, 58–66.

Glenn, J. K., Lawler, F. H., & Hoerl, M. S. (1987). Physician referrals in a competitive environment: An estimate of the economic impact of a referral. *Journal of the American Medical Association, 258*, 1920–1923.

Glenn, M. L. (1985). Toward collaborative family-oriented health care. *Family Systems Medicine, 3*, 466–475.

Goffman, E. (1974). *Frame analysis: An essay on the organization of experience*. Cambridge, MA: Harvard University Press.

Goffman, E. (1981). Replies and responses. In E. Goffman (Ed.), *Forms of talk* (pp. 52–77). Philadelphia: University of Pennsylvania Press.

Goldfield, N., Neinstein, L., & Wohlgelernter, D. (1986). Cardiovascular evaluation of adolescents and young adults: Salient aspects of the examination. *Postgraduate Medicine, 79*, 111–118.

Good Housekeeping family health & medical guide. (1979). Des Moines, IN: Hearst Corporation.

Good, M-J. D., Good, B. J., & Cleary, P. D. (1987). Do patients attitudes influence physician recognition of psychosocial problems in primary care? *Journal of Family Practice, 25*, 53–59.

Green, M., & Solnit, A. J. (1964). Reactions to the threatened loss of a child: A vulnerable child syndrome—Pediatric management of the dying child, Part III. *Pediatrics, 34*, 58–66.

Greenberg, L. C. (1989). Book review of *The state of the art in family therapy research*. *Journal of Marital and Family Therapy, 15*, 207–208.

Gulich, E., & Quasthoff, U. M. (Eds). (1986a). Narrative analysis: An interdisciplinary dialogue [Special issue]. *Poetics, 15*.

Gulich, E., & Quasthoff, U. M. (1986b). Story-telling in conversation: Cognitive and interactive aspects. *Poetics, 15*, 217–241.

Hansen, J. P., Bobula, J., Meyer, D., Kusher, K., & Pridham, K. (1987). Treat or refer: Patients' interest in family physician involvement in their psychosocial problems. *Journal of Family Practice, 24*, 499–503.

Hansen, J. P., Brown, S. E., Sullivan, Jr., R. J., & Muhlbaier, L. H. (1982). Factors related to an effective referral and consultation process. *Journal of Family Practice, 15*, 651–656.

Hein, N., & Wodak, R. (1987). Medical interviews in internal medicine: Some results of an empirical investigation. *Text, 7*, 37–65.

Helman, C. G. (1985). Communication in primary care: The role of the patient and practitioner explanatory models. *Social Science and Medicine, 20*, 923–931.

Hersher, L. (1988). Avoiding anxiety about 'innocent' heart murmur. *American Journal of Diseases of Children, 142*, 586–587.

Hewitt, J. P., & Stokes, R. (1975). Disclaimers. *American Sociological Review, 40*, 1–11.

Hopper, R. (1988). Speech, for instance. The exemplar in studies of conversation. *Journal of Language and Social Psychology, 7*, 47–63.

Hull, F. M. (1987). The role of socio-behavioural scientists in health care practice. Social *Science & Medicine, 25*, 679–687.

Jick, T. D. (1983). Mixing qualitative and quantitative methods: Triangulation in action. In J. Van Maanen (Ed.), *Qualitative methodology* (pp. 135–147). Beverly Hills, CA: Sage Publications.

Keeney, B. P. (1983). *Aesthetics of change*. New York: Guilford Press.

Keeney, B. P. (1987a). The construction of therapeutic realities. *Psychotherapy, 24*, 469–476.

Keeney, B. P. (1987b). *Recursive frame analysis: Class notes*. Unpublished manuscript, Texas Tech University, Department of Human Development and Family Studies, Lubbock, TX.

Keeney, B. P. (1988). Autonomy in dialogue. *Irish Journal of Psychology, 9*, 101–109.

Keeney, B. P. (1990a). *Improvisional therapy: A practical guide for creative clinical strategies*. St. Paul, MN: Systemic Therapy Press. (Available from Systemic Therapy Press, 1946 Laurel Avenue, St. Paul, MN 55104)

Keeney, B. P. (1990b). Recursive frame analysis: A method for organizing therapeutic discourse. *Therapia Familiare, 33*, 25–39.

Keeney, B. P., & Bobele, M. (1989). A brief note on family violence. *Australian and New Zealand Journal of Family Therapy, 10*, 93–95.

Keeney, B. K., & Morris, J. P. (1985a). Family therapy practice and research: A dialogue. In L. L. Andreozzi (Ed.), *Integrating research and clinical practice* (pp. 98–107). Rockville, MD: Aspen Systems Corporation.

Keeney, B. P., & Morris, J. P. (1985b). Implications of cybernetic epistemology for clinical research: A reply to Howard. *Journal of Counseling and Development, 63*, 548–550.

Keeney, B. P., & Ross, J. M. (1985). *Mind in therapy: Constructing systemic family therapies*. New York: Basic Books.

Keeney, B. P., & Silverstein, O. (1986). *The therapeutic voice of Olga Silverstein*. New York: Guilford Press.

Keppel, G. (1982). *Design and analysis: A researcher's handbook* (2nd ed.). Engelwood Cliffs, NJ: Prentice-Hall.

Kerlinger, F. N. (1986). *Foundations of behavioral research* (3rd ed.). New York: Holt, Rinehart and Winston.

Kiester, Jr., E. (Ed.). (1982). *Better Homes and Gardens new family medical guide*. Des Moines, IA: Meredith Corporation.

Kosa, J., Alpert, J., & Haggerty, R. J. (1967). On the reliability of family health information: A comparative study of mothers' reports on illness and related behavior. *Social Science & Medicine, 1*, 165–181.

Kreps, G. L., & Thornton, B. C. (1984). *Health communication: Theory and practice*. New York: Longman.

Kunz, J. R. M., & Finkel, A. J. (Eds.). (1987). *The American Medical Association family medical guide* (rev. ed. and updated). New York: Random House.

Labov, W., & Fanshel, D. (1977). *Therapeutic discourse: Psychotherapy as conversation*. New York: Academic Press.

Lakoff, G., & Ross, J. R. (1979). Preamble to the series. In A. L. Becker & A. A.

Yengoyan (Ed.), *The imagination of reality: Essays in Southeast Asian coherence systems* (pp. vii–viii). Norwood, NJ: Ablex.

Lather, P. (1986). Research as praxis. *Harvard Educational Review, 56*, 257–277.

Leeds-Hurwitz, W. (1987). The social history of the natural history of an interview: A multidisciplinary investigation of social communication. *Research on Language and Social Interaction*, 20, 1–51.

Linde, C. (1986). Private stories in public discourse: Narrative analysis in the social sciences. *Poetics, 15*, 183–202.

Linde, L. M., Rasof, B., Dunn, O. J., & Rabb, E. (1966). Attitudinal factors in congenital heart disease. *Pediatrics, 38*, 92–101.

Lyne, J. (1985). Rhetorics of inquiry. *Quarterly Journal of Speech, 71*, 65–73.

Mackenzie, T. B. (1982). The initial patient interview: Identifying when psychosocial factors are at work. *Postgraduate Medicine, 74*, 259–265.

Mahrer, A. R. (1988). Discovery-oriented psychotherapy research: Rational, aims, and methods. *American Psychologist, 43*, 694–702.

Maisede, P. (1987). The permanent text construction: A neglected dimension of therapeutic discourse. *Text, 7*, 67–87.

Mathews, J. J. (1983). The communication process in clinical settings. *Social Science and Medicine, 17*, 1371–1378.

McDaniel, S. H., Bank, J., Campbell, T., Mancini, J., & Shore, B. (1986). Using groups as a consultant: A systems approach to medical care. In L. C. Wynne, S. H. McDaniel, & T. T. Weber (Eds.), *Systems consultation: A new perspective for family therapy* (pp. 181–198). New York: Guilford Press.

McNamara, D. G. (1987a). *Innocent Heart Murmurs: Information for Parents and Patients.* (Available from Dr. Dan G. McNamara at Texas Children's Hospital, 6621 Fannin St., Houston, TX 77030)

McNamara, D. G. (1987b). The pediatrician and the innocent heart murmur. *American Journal of Diseases of Children, 141*, 1161.

McNamara, D. G. (1988). In reply to "Avoiding anxiety about 'innocent' heart murmur". *American Journal of Diseases of Children, 142*, 587.

McQuown, N. A. (1971a). Chapter 10: Summary, conclusion, and outlook. In N. A. McQuown (Ed.), *The natural history of an interview* (pp. 1–10). (Available from Microfilm Collection of Manuscripts on Cultural Anthropology. Chicago: University of Chicago, Joseph Regenstein Library, Department of Photoduplication)

McQuown, N. A. (1971b). Forword. In N. A. McQuown (Ed.), *The natural history of an interview* (pp. 1–5). (Available from Microfilm Collection of Manuscripts on Cultural Anthropology. Chicago: University of Chicago, Joseph Regenstein Library, Department of Photoduplication)

McQuown, N. A. (Ed.). (1971c). *The natural history of an interview*. (Available from Microfilm Collection of Manuscripts on Cultural Anthropology. Chicago: University of Chicago, Joseph Regenstein Library, Department of Photoduplication)

Meador, C. K. (1965). The art and science of nondisease. *New England Journal of Medicine, 272*, 92–95.

Mishler, E. G. (1979). Meaning in context: Is there any other kind? *Harvard Educational Review, 49*, 1–19.

Montalvo, B., Schor, E. L., & Moore, M. (1987). Psychosocial aspects of pediatrics: Middle-level theory building. *Family Systems Medicine*, 5, 65–78.

Morrell, D. C., Evans, M. E., Morris, R. W., & Roland, M. O. (1986). The "five minute" consultation: Effects of time constraint on clinical content and patient satisfaction. *British Medical Journal, 292*, 870–873.

Munson, S. (1986). Family-oriented consultation in pediatrics. In L. C. Wynne, S. H. McDaniel, & T. T. Weber (Eds.), *Systems consultation: A new perspective for family therapy* (pp. 219–239). New York: Guilford Press.

Nelson, J. S., Megill, A., & McCloskey, D. N. (1988). *The rhetoric of the human sciences: Language and arguement in scholarship and public affairs*. Madison, WI: University of Wisconsin Press.

Niklas, D. (1982). Methodological controversies between social and medical sciences. *Social Science & Medicine, 16*, 659–665.

Papert, S. (1980). *Mindstorms: Children, computers, and powerful ideas*. New York: Basic Books.

Paraskos, J. A. (1988). The innocent murmur. *Hospital Practice, 23*, 20–29.

Park, J. M., Maddux, J. E., & Sridaromont, S. (1983). *Psychological aspects of children with heart defects and their families*. Unpublished manuscript, Texas Tech University Health Sciences Center, Department of Pediatrics, Lubbock, TX.

Park, J. M., Sridaromont, S., Schmer, V., Stormberg, J., Douthit, P. E., Gale, J., & Chenail, R. (1988). *Psychosocial aspects of children with heart defects and their children*. Unpublished manuscript, Texas Tech University Health Sciences Center, Department of Pediatrics and Texas Tech University, Department of Human Development and Family Studies, Lubbock, TX.

Peck, B. B. (1974). Physical medicine and family dynamics: The dialectics of rehabilitation. *Family Process*, 13, 469–480.

Phoenix, V. G., & Lindeman, M. L. (1982). Language and therapeutic change. In R. J. Di Pietro (Ed.), *Linguistics and the professions: Proceedings of the second annual Delaware symposium on language studies* (pp. 3–25). Norwood, NJ: Ablex.

Pittenger, R. E., Hockett, C. F., & Danehy, J. J. (1960). *The first five minutes: A sample of microscopic interview analysis*. Ithaca, NY: Paul Martineau.

Potter, J., & Wetherell, M. (1987). *Discourse and social psychology: Beyond attitudes and behavior*. Beverly Hills, CA: Sage Publications.

Pluckham, M. (1978). *Human communication: The matrix of nursing*. New York: McGraw-Hill.

Prince, E., Frader, J., & Bosk, C. (1982). On hedging in physician-physician discourse. In R. J. Di Pietro (Ed.), *Linguistics and the professions: Proceedings of the second annual Delaware symposium on language studies* (pp. 83–97). Norwood, NJ: Ablex.

Raimbault, G., Cachin, O., Limal, J-M., Eliacheff, C., & Rappaport, R. (1975). Aspects of communication between patients and doctors: An analysis of the discourse in medical interviews. *Pediatrics*, 55, 401–405.

Rawlins, W. K. (1987). Gregory Bateson and the composition of human communication. *Research on Language and Social Interaction, 20*, 53–77.

Ricoeur, P. (1981). The narrative function. In J. B. Thompson (Ed. and Trans.), *Paul Ricoeur: Hermeneutics and the human sciences: Essays on language, action and interpretation* (pp. 274–296). Cambridge, England: Cambridge University Press. (Reprinted from *Etudes Theologiques et Religieuses*, 1979, 54, 209–230)

Rinaldi, R. (1985). Positive effects of psychosocial interventions on total health care: A review of the literature. *Family Systems Medicine, 3*, 417–426.

Rogers, T. F. (1987). Improving the fit between social science and health care practice: Suggested next steps for the researcher. *Social Science & Medicine, 25*, 689–696.

Roland, M. O., Bartholomew, J., Courtenay, M. J. F., Morris, R. W., & Morrell, D. C. (1986). The "five minute" consultation: Effect of time constraint on verbal communication. *British Medical Journal, 292*, 874–876.

Sargent, J. (1985). Physician-family therapist collaboration: Children with medical problems. *Family Systems Medicine, 3*, 454–465.

Scheflen, A. E. (1973). *Communicational structure: Analysis of a psychotherapy transaction*. Bloomington, IN: Indiana University Press.

Schumacher, J. A. (1989). *Human posture: The nature of inquiry*. Albany, NY: State University of New York Press.

Schwartz, H., & Jacobs, J. (1979). *Qualitative sociology: A method to the madness*. New York: Free Press.

Schwartzman, J. (1985). Health, illness, and the family: An evolutionary perspective. *Family Systems Medicine, 3*, 454–465.

Schwenk, T. L. (1987). Caring about and caring for the psychosocial needs of patients. *Journal of Family Practice, 24*, 461–463.

Scott, M. B., & Lyman, S. M. (1968). Accounts. *American Sociological Review, 33*, 46–62.

Shuy, R. W. (1984). Linguistics in other fields. In B. J. Siegal, A. R. Beals, & S. A. Tyler (Eds.), *Annual Review of Anthropology* (Vol. 13) (pp. 419–445). Palo Alto, CA: Annual Reviews.

Siebert, C. (1990, February). The rehumanization of the heart: What doctors have forgotten, poets have always known. *Harper's Magazine*, pp. 53–60.

Simon, F. B., Stierlin, H., & Wynne, L. C. (1985). *The language of family therapy: A systemic vocabulary and sourcebook*. New York: Family Process Press.

Spence, D. P. (1982). *Narrative truth and historical truth: Meaning and interpretation in psychoanalysis*. New York: W. W. Norton.

Spence, D. P. (1987). *The Freudian metaphor: Toward paradigm change in psychoanalysis*. New York: W. W. Norton.

Spencer-Brown, G. (1972). *Laws of form*. New York: E. P. Dutton

Stein, H. F., & Pontious, J. M. (1985). Family and beyond: The larger context of noncompliance. *Family Systems Medicine, 3*, 179–189.

Stokes, R., & Hewitt, J. P. (1976). Aligning actions. *American Sociological Review, 41*, 838–849.

Stone, G. C. (1979). Patient compliance and the role of the expert. *Journal of Social Issues, 35*, 34–59.

Street, Jr., R. L. (1986). Interaction processes and outcomes in interviews. In M. L. McLaughlin (Ed.), *Communication yearbook 9* (pp. 215–250). Beverly Hills, CA: Sage.

Street, Jr., R. L., & Wiemann, J. M. (1987). Patient satisfaction with physicians' interpersonal involvement, expressiveness, and dominance. In M. L. McLaughlin (Ed.), *Communication yearbook 10* (pp. 591–612). Newbury Park, CA: Sage.

Szasz, T. S., & Hollender, M. H. (1956). A contribution to the philosophy of medicine: The basic models of the doctor-patient relationship. *American Medical Association Archives of Internal Medicine, 97*, 585–592.

Tannen, D. (1979). What's in a frame? Surface evidence for underlying expectations. In R. O. Freedle (Ed.), *New directions in discourse processing* (Vol. 2, pp. 137–181). Norwood, NJ: Ablex.

Tannen, D., & Wallat, C. (1983). Doctor/mother/child communication: Linguistic analysis of a pediatric interaction. In S, Fisher & A. D. Todd (Eds.), *The social organization of doctor-patient communication* (pp. 203–219). Washington, DC: Center for Applied Linguistics.

Tannen, D., & Wallat, C. (1986). Medical professionals and parents: A linguistic analysis of communication across contexts. *Language in Society, 15*, 295–312.

Todd, A. D. (1984). The prescription of contraception: Negotiations between doctors and patients. *Discourse Processes, 7*, 171–200.

Tracy, K. (1988). A discourse analysis of four discourse studies. *Discourse Processes, 11*, 243–259.

Troemel-Ploetz, S. (1977). "She is just not an open person.": A linguistic analysis of a restructuring intervention in family therapy. *Family Process, 16*, 339–352.

Tyler, S. A. (1986). Post-modern ethnography: From document of the occult to occult document. In J. Clifford & G. E. Marcus (Eds.), *Writing culture: The poetics and politics of ethnography* (pp. 122–140). Berkeley, CA: University of California Press.

Urmson, J. O., & Sbisa, M. (Eds.). (1975). *How to do things with words* (2nd ed.). Cambridge, MA: Harvard University Press.

von Foerster, H. (1984a). On constructing a reality. In P. Watzlawick (Ed.), *The invented reality: How do we know what we believe we know? (Contributions to constructivism)* (pp. 41–61). New York: W. W. Norton.

von Foerster, H. (1984b). Principles of self-organization in a socio-managerial context. In H. Ulrich & G. J. B. Probst (Eds.), *Self-organization and management of social systems: Insights, promises, doubts, and questions* (pp. 2–24). New York: Springer-Verlag.

Wadsworth, M. (1976). Studies of doctor-patient communication. In M. Wadsworth & D. Robinson (Eds.), *Studies in everyday medical life* (pp. 3–12). London: Martin Robertson.

Waitzkin, H. (1984). Doctor-patient communication: Clinical implications of social scientific research. *Journal of the American Medical Association, 252*, 2441–2446.

Waitzkin, H. (1985). Information giving in medical care. *Journal of Health and Social Behavior, 26*, 81–101.

Wasserman, R. C., Inui, T. S. (1983). Systematic analysis of clinical-patient interactions: A critique of recent approaches with suggestions for future research. *Medical Care, 21*, 279–293.

Watzlawick, P. (1984). Effect or cause? In P. Watzlawick (Ed.), *The invented reality: How do we know what we believe we know? (Contributions to constructivism)* (pp. 62–68). New York: W. W. Norton.

Webb, B., & Stimson, G. (1976). People's accounts of medical encounters. In M. Wadsworth & D. Robinson (Eds.), *Studies in everyday medical life* (pp. 108–122). London: Martin Robertson.

Wellisch, D. K., & Cohen, M. M. (1986). The family therapist as systems consultant to medical oncology. In L. C. Wynne, S. H. McDaniel, & T. T. Weber (Eds.), *Systems consultation: A new perspective for family therapy* (pp. 199–218). New York: Guilford Press.

West, C. (1984). Medical misfires: Mishearings, misgivings, and misunderstandings in the physician-patient dialogues. *Discourse Processes, 7*, 107–134.

Wiedemann, P. M. (1986). Don't tell any stories: Theories and discoveries concerning story-telling in the therapeutic setting. *Poetics, 15*, 43–56.

Wodak, R. (1981). How do I put my problem? Problem presentation in therapy and interview. *Text, 1*, 191–213.

Wodak, R. (1986). Tales from the Vienna woods: Sociolinguistic and psycholinguistic considerations of narrative analysis. *Poetics, 15* 153–182.

Worobey, J., O'Hair, D., & O'Hair, M. J. C. (1987). Pediatrician-patient-parent communications: A descriptive analysis. *Language & Communication, 7*, 293–301.

Wynne, L. C. (1988). An overview of the state of the art: What should be expected in current family therapy research. In L. C. Wynne (Ed.), *The state of the art in family therapy research: Controversies and recommendations* (pp. 249–280). New York: Family Process Press.

Yaffe, M. J., & Stewart, M. A. (1986). Patients' attitudes to the relevance of nonmedical problems in family medicine care. *Journal of Family Practice, 23*, 241–244.

Author Index

V

W

Y

Subject Index

K

L

M

N

O

P

R

S

T

V

W

Y